ORTHOPEDIC CLINICS OF NORTH AMERICA

www.orthopedic.theclinics.com

Common Complications in Orthopedic Surgery

July 2021 • Volume 52 • Number 3

Editor-in-Chief

FREDERICK M. AZAR

Editorial Board

MICHAEL J. BEEBE
CLAYTON C. BETTIN
TYLER J. BROLIN
JAMES H. CALANDRUCCIO
BENJAMIN J. GREAR
BENJAMIN M. MAUCK
WILLIAM M. MIHALKO
BENJAMIN SHEFFER
DAVID D. SPENCE
PATRICK C. TOY
JOHN C. WEINLEIN

ELSEVIER

1600 John F. Kennedy Boulevard • Suite 1800 • Philadelphia, Pennsylvania, 19103-2899.

http://www.orthopedic.theclinics.com

ORTHOPEDIC CLINICS OF NORTH AMERICA Volume 52, Number 3
July 2021 ISSN 0030-5898, ISBN-13: 978-0-323-89672-6

Editor: Lauren Boyle
Developmental Editor: Ann Gielou Posedio

Orthopedic Clinics of North America (ISSN 0030-5898) is published quarterly by Elsevier Inc., 360 Park Avenue South, New York, NY 10010-1710. Months of issue are January, April, July, and October. Business and Editorial Offices: 1600 John F. Kennedy Blvd., Suite 1800, Philadelphia, PA 19103-2899. Customer Service Office: 3251 Riverport Lane, Maryland Heights, MO 63043. Periodicals postage paid at New York, NY and additional mailing offices. Subscription prices are $347.00 per year for (US individuals), $1,003.00 per year for (US institutions), $411.00 per year (Canadian individuals), $1,028.00 per year (Canadian institutions), $476.00 per year (international individuals), $1,028.00 per year (international institutions), $100.00 per year (US students), $100.00 per year for (Canadian students), $220.00 per year for (international students). Foreign air speed delivery is included in all *Clinics* subscription prices. All prices are subject to change without notice. **POSTMASTER:** Send change of address to *Orthopedic Clinics of North America*, **Elsevier Health Sciences Division, Subscription Customer Service, 3251 Riverport Lane, Maryland Heights, MO 63043. Customer Service (orders, claims, online, change of address): Elsevier Health Sciences Division, Subscription Customer Service, 3251 Riverport Lane, Maryland Heights, MO 63043. Tel: 1-800-654-2452 (U.S. and Canada); 314-447-8871 (outside U.S. and Canada). Fax: 314-447-8029. E-mail:** journalscustomerservice-usa@elsevier.com **(for print support);** journalsonlinesupport-usa@elsevier.com **(for online support).**

Reprints. For copies of 100 or more, of articles in this publication, please contact the Commercial Reprints Department, Elsevier Inc., 360 Park Avenue South, New York, NY 10010-1710. Tel.: 212-633-3874; Fax: 212-633-3820; E-mail: reprints@elsevier.com.

Orthopedic Clinics of North America is covered in MEDLINE/PubMed (Index Medicus), Cinahl, Excerpta Medica, and Cumulative Index to Nursing and Allied Health Literature.

EDITORIAL BOARD

CONTRIBUTORS

AUTHORS

JOHN G. ANDERSON, MD
Orthopaedic Associates of Michigan, Grand
Rapids, Michigan

JASON BARITEAU, MD
Associate Professor, Department of
Orthopaedic Surgery, Emory University School
of Medicine, Atlanta, Georgia

DONALD R. BOHAY, MD, FACS
Orthopaedic Associates of Michigan, Grand
Rapids, Michigan

KELSEY BONILLA, MD
Resident, Department of Orthopaedics,
University of Pennsylvania, Philadelphia,
Pennsylvania

MICHELLE COLEMAN, MD/PhD
Assistant Professor, Department of
Orthopaedic Surgery, Emory University School
of Medicine, Atlanta, Georgia

EILEEN M. COLLITON, MD
Department of Orthopaedic Surgery, Tufts
Medical Center, Boston, Massachusetts

JOSEPH T. CLINE, MD
Orthopaedic Surgery Resident, Department of
Orthopaedic Surgery and Biomedical
Engineering, University of Tennessee-
Campbell Clinic, Memphis, Tennessee

TRAVIS A. DOERING, MD
Department of Orthopaedic Surgery and
Biomedical Engineering, University of
Tennessee-Campbell Clinic, Memphis,
Tennessee

DEREK DONEGAN, MD, MBA
Assistant Professor of Orthopaedic Surgery,
Department of Orthoapedics, Division of
Orthopaedic Trauma, University of
Pennsylvania, Philadelphia, Pennsylvania

DANIEL F. DRAKE, MD
Fellow, Department of Orthopedic Surgery,
Akron Children's Hospital, Akron, Ohio

TSOLA A. EFEJUKU, BSA
School of Medicine, The University of Texas
Medical Branch, Galveston, Texas

TRAVIS R. FLICK, MD
Research Fellow, Department of Orthopaedic
Surgery, Tulane University School of Medicine,
New Orleans, Louisiana

HAYDEN S. HOLBROOK, MD
Department of Orthopaedic Surgery and
Biomedical Engineering, University of
Tennessee-Campbell Clinic, Memphis,
Tennessee

ANDREW JAWA, MD
Department of Orthopaedic Surgery, New
England Baptist Hospital, Boston,
Massachusetts; Boston Sports and Shoulder
Center, Waltham, Massachusetts

RISHIN KADAKIA, MD
Assistant Professor, Department of
Orthopaedic Surgery, Emory University School
of Medicine, Atlanta, Georgia

JACOB M. KIRSCH, MD
Department of Orthopaedic Surgery, New
England Baptist Hospital, Boston,
Massachusetts; Boston Sports and Shoulder
Center, Waltham, Massachusetts

MATTHEW LUNATI, MD
Department of Orthopaedic Surgery, Emory
University School of Medicine, Atlanta,
Georgia

KARIM MAHMOUD, MD
Department of Orthopaedic Surgery, Emory
University School of Medicine, Atlanta,
Georgia

BENJAMIN M. MAUCK, MD
Department of Orthopaedic Surgery and Biomedical Engineering, University of Tennessee-Campbell Clinic, Memphis, Tennessee

SAMUEL GRAY MCCLATCHY, MD
Orthopaedic Surgery Resident, Department of Orthopaedic Surgery and Biomedical Engineering, University of Tennessee-Campbell Clinic, Memphis, Tennessee

WILLIAM M. MIHALKO, MD, PhD
J.R. Hyde Professor and Chair Joint Graduate Program in Biomedical Engineering, Department of Orthopaedic Surgery and Biomedical Engineering, University of Tennessee- Campbell Clinic, Memphis, Tennessee

KEVIN H. PHAN, MD
Orthopaedic Associates of Michigan, Grand Rapids, Michigan

ZACHARY K. PHARR, MD
Orthopaedic Surgery Resident, Department of Orthopaedic Surgery and Biomedical Engineering, University of Tennessee-Campbell Clinic, Memphis, Tennessee

CARSON M. RIDER, MD
Orthopaedic Surgery Resident, Department of Orthopaedic Surgery and Biomedical Engineering, University of Tennessee-Campbell Clinic, Memphis, Tennessee

TODD F. RITZMAN, MD
Chair, Department of Orthopedic Surgery, Akron Children's Hospital, Akron, Ohio

BAILEY J. ROSS, BA
MS3, Department of Orthopaedic Surgery, Tulane University School of Medicine, New Orleans, Louisiana

WILLIAM F. SHERMAN, MD, MBA
Associate Professor, Adult Reconstruction Hip/Knee, Research Fellowship Director, Department of Orthopaedic Surgery, Tulane University School of Medicine, New Orleans, Louisiana

JEREMY S. SOMERSON, MD
Assistant Professor of Orthopaedic Surgery, Department of Orthopaedic Surgery and Rehabilitation, The University of Texas Medical Branch, Galveston, Texas

MATTHEW SULLIVAN, MD
Assistant Professor of Orthopaedic Surgery, Chief of Orthopaedic Trauma Division, SUNY Upstate, East Syracuse, New York

NORFLEET B. THOMPSON, MD
Department of Orthopaedic Surgery and Biomedical Engineering, University of Tennessee-Campbell Clinic, Memphis, Tennessee

THOMAS W. THROCKMORTON, MD
Professor, Department of Orthopaedic Surgery and Biomedical Engineering, University of Tennessee-Campbell Clinic, Memphis, Tennessee

PATRICK C. TOY, MD
Associate Professor, Department of Orthopaedic Surgery and Biomedical Engineering, University of Tennessee-Campbell Clinic, Memphis, Tennessee

PAUL J. WEATHERBY, MD
Department of Orthopaedic Surgery and Rehabilitation, The University of Texas Medical Branch, Galveston, Texas

ANDREW J. WODOWSKI, MD
OrthoSouth, Memphis, Tennessee

CONTENTS

Knee and Hip Reconstruction

Instability remains the leading cause of reoperation following total hip arthroplasty (THA). In this article, the risk factors for instability after THA are reviewed,
including patient-related characteristics, surgical techniques, positioning of implants, and the role of advanced technology and robotics as a platform that
may reduce the incidence of instability.

Based on a series of 407 outpatient total hip arthroplasties performed by a single surgeon, a standardized protocol for blood loss management in outpatient
arthroplasty was developed consisting of a presurgical hematocrit of greater
than 36%, administration of tranexamic acid, prophylactic introduction of albumin, hypotensive epidural anesthesia, monopolar electrocautery, and bipolar
sealer. This protocol uses techniques that alone are not novel but together
create a standardized and reproducible pathway that when implemented can
increase the safety of outpatient hip arthroplasty.

This study compares anterior supine intermuscular total hip arthroplasty performed at an ambulatory surgery center with the same procedure performed in
a hospital setting in regard to complications and costs. The ambulatory surgery
center had significantly shorter postoperative stays and superior visual analog
pain scores at 3 months. No differences were noted in operative time, blood
loss, or complications. Costs were significantly different between groups, with
significant cost savings noted in the ambulatory surgery center group.

Trauma

Rotational malreduction is a common yet underreported postoperative complication following intramedullary nailing of long bone fractures. In most situations,
this can be prevented at the time of initial surgery with meticulous preoperative
planning, careful use of intraoperative fluoroscopy, and awareness of risk factors
for malrotation. However, rotational alignment remains difficult to assess by clinical examination so a high index of suspicion is always necessary. Here, the authors review the literature on this complication and report on 3 such cases of
femoral and the tibial malrotation, methods for calculating femoral version and
tibial torsion, and techniques for correcting these deformities.

Pediatrics

Despite advances in surgical techniques and technology, casting remains an important treatment modality in the armamentarium of orthopedic surgery. Opportunities for skill development and complication management are a decreasing commodity for the surgeon in training. Appropriate indications for casting and technical expertise of cast application are key to complication avoidance. Prompt recognition and evaluation of potential complications are key to optimizing patient outcomes. Following the lead of the American Board of Orthopedic Surgery Resident Skills Modules, we implore teaching institutions to develop and maintain robust teaching programs, skills acquisitions laboratories, and assessments for confirmation of competency for all residency programs.

Hand and Wrist

Distal radial fractures are associated with good outcomes; however, although they occur at low rates, complications can significantly impair treatment success. Therefore, the treating surgeon should be aware of potential complications associated with each treatment type and how to best prevent them. Although certain patient-specific and fracture-specific factors may increase the risk of adverse outcomes, most are nonmodifiable risk factors at the time of presentation, so it is imperative that every effort is made to mitigate these risk factors to prevent long-term morbidity. Patients should be well-informed about these complications and potential symptoms so that they can be addressed expeditiously.

Although the overall complication rate of volar plating approaches 15%, less than 5% require reoperation. Certain factors involving the patient, the fracture, and/or the surgeon may affect the overall complication risk. Patient factors, including body mass index greater than 35 and diabetes mellitus, may increase complication risk with volar plating, but older patient age does not seem to significantly alter risk.

Shoulder and Elbow

Reverse total shoulder arthroplasty (RSA) continues to see tremendous growth as the indications have expanded. A variety of complications have been described, including fractures of the acromion or scapular spine. These fractures are painful and can compromise shoulder stability and functional outcomes following RSA. Multiple studies have recently investigated the incidence, risk factors, and treatment strategies for these injuries. In this article, the authors review current literature and discuss the incidence, cause, associated risk factors, treatment options, and outcomes following fractures of the acromion or scapular spine after RSA.

For practicing shoulder arthroplasty surgeons, it is advisable to consider a breadth of data sources concerning complications and outcomes. Although published series from high-volume centers are the primary source of data, these results may not be generalizable to a wide range of practice settings. National or health system–specific registry and medical device databases are useful adjuncts to assess the changing complication profile of shoulder arthroplasty, as well as to understand the complications specific to certain implants or implant types. To reduce the risk of postoperative complications, surgeons must have a clear understanding of the most common modes of failure.

Foot and Ankle

Outpatient orthopedic surgery is gradually becoming the standard across the country, as it has been found to significantly lower costs without compromising patient care. Peripheral nerve blocks (PNBs) are largely what have made this transition possible by providing patients excellent pain control in the immediate postoperative period. However, with the increasing use of PNBs, it is important to recognize that they are not without complications. Although rare, these complications can cause patients a significant amount of morbidity. It is important for surgeons to know the risks of peripheral nerve blocks and to inform their patients.

Hallux rigidus is the most common arthritic pathology of the foot. This review article discusses the pathophysiology and common clinical presentation of hallux rigidus. Furthermore, we discuss multiple classification systems that categorize the arthritic process and guide management. Surgical interventions include cheilectomy, Moberg osteotomy, synthetic cartilage implants, interpositional arthroplasty, and arthrodesis. The common complications are reviewed, and the rates of these complications highlighted. Surgical options for hallux rigidus globally have successful outcomes with low rates of complications when done on appropriate patients.

COMMON COMPLICATIONS IN ORTHOPEDIC SURGERY

PREFACE

Despite an appropriate choice of treatment, careful preoperative planning, and meticulous technique, complications can occur. This issue describes some of the possible complications of orthopedic treatment and provides information on how to avoid them.

Dr Flick and colleagues describe risk factors for instability after total hip arthroplasty (THA) and discuss the role of advanced technology and robotics as a platform that may lower the frequency of instability. Dr McClatchy and colleagues present a standardized protocol for blood loss management in outpatient THA that can increase the safety of outpatient hip arthroplasty. In a comparison of safety and cost-effectiveness of THA in an ambulatory surgical center to those in a hospital, Dr Wodowski and colleagues report significantly shorter postoperative stays, superior visual analog pain scores at 3 months, and significant cost savings with THA in an ambulatory surgery center, with no differences in operative time, blood loss, or complications.

Rotational malreduction is a common yet underreported postoperative complication of intramedullary nailing of long bone fractures. Dr Sullivan and colleagues emphasize that prevention at the time of initial surgery involves meticulous preoperative planning, careful use of intraoperative fluoroscopy, and awareness of risk factors for malrotation. They also describe techniques for correcting malrotation deformities.

As noted by Drs Drake and Ritzman, not all complications are associated with operative treatment. They describe appropriate indications for casting and technical expertise of cast application as key factors in complication avoidance in pediatric patients. Prompt recognition and evaluation of potential complications are noted to be key to optimizing patient outcomes. They recommend that teaching institutions develop and maintain robust teaching programs, skills acquisitions laboratories, and assessments for confirmation of casting competency for all residency programs.

Distal radial fractures are among the most common upper-extremity fractures, and their treatment can be fraught with complications. Dr Holbrook and colleagues describe complications that can occur with different treatment types and how to best prevent them. Dr Thompson focuses on complications that can occur with volar plating of distal radial fractures, noting certain factors involving the patient, the fracture, and/or the surgeon that may affect the overall complication risk.

Complications that may occur with anatomic total shoulder arthroplasty and with reverse shoulder arthroplasty are described and discussed by Dr Colliton and colleagues and Dr Weatherby and colleagues. Dr Colliton and colleagues discuss the incidence, cause, associated risk factors, treatment options, and outcomes following fractures of the acromion or scapular spine after reverse shoulder arthroplasty, while Dr Weatherby and colleagues describe the leading causes of failure after anatomic shoulder arthroplasty and complications specific to certain implants or implant types.

Dr Phan and colleagues note that although peripheral nerve blocks are widely used in outpatient foot and ankle surgery, they are not without complications that can cause a significant amount of morbidity. In their review of hallux rigidus management, Dr Lunati and colleagues discuss the pathophysiology and common clinical presentation of hallux rigidus and review rates of common complications.

Overall, this issue provides much useful information about common complications that can occur with treatment of orthopedic conditions. We hope this information will be useful to guide you when caring for your patients and will help you avoid these complications.

Frederick M. Azar, MD
Department of Orthopaedic Surgery &
Biomedical Engineering
University of Tennessee–Campbell Clinic
1211 Union Avenue, Suite 510
Memphis, TN 38104, USA

E-mail address:
fazar@campbellclinic.com

Orthop Clin N Am 52 (2021) xi
https://doi.org/10.1016/j.ocl.2021.03.012
0030-5898/21/© 2021 Published by Elsevier Inc.

Knee and Hip Reconstruction

Instability After Total Hip Arthroplasty and the Role of Advanced and Robotic Technology

Travis R. Flick, MD[a], Bailey J. Ross, BA[a],
William F. Sherman, MD, MBA[b],*

KEYWORDS

- Total hip arthroplasty • Instability • Robotics • Risk factors • Component position

KEY POINTS

- Modifiable risk factors for instability following total hip arthroplasty include tobacco use, alcohol abuse, and obesity. Factors such as increased age, prior hip surgery, and reduced spinopelvic mobility are nonmodifiable.
- Surgical factors increasing the risk of instability include use of a posterior approach and acetabular component placement with a vertically displaced center of rotation.
- Implant factors that improve hip stability include larger femoral head sizes, high-offset stems, dual-mobility implants, and elevated/lipped liners during posterior approaches.
- Spinopelvic imaging is a key component of preoperative risk stratification and aids physicians in developing individualized operative plans that mitigate risk of instability.

BACKGROUND

Total hip arthroplasty (THA) has been revolutionary in improving quality of life for patients with end-stage osteoarthritis.[1] As one of the most successful orthopedic surgeries, THA has a survivorship of more than 95% at 10 years and patient satisfaction of as high as 93%.[2–4] Hip instability is one of the most frequent complications encountered, with a reported incidence of 0.3% to 10% after primary THA.[5–7] More importantly, instability remains the inciting factor in more than 22% of all revision THAs.[8] Because the annual volume of THA performed in America is projected to increase to 572,000 by 2030, with a consequential increase in incident prosthetic dislocations,[9,10] it is paramount to continue developing techniques to mitigate instability. This article reviews the risk factors for instability after THA and the role advanced technology and robotics can have in reducing the incidence of instability after primary THA.

PREOPERATIVE RISK FACTORS

Modifiable Patient Risk Factors

Tobacco use is a strong risk factor for early instability and aseptic loosening following THA.[11] Although the exact mechanism is unclear, tobacco use seems to disrupt bone healing and osteointegration of the prosthetic implant.[12,13] Several studies have also reported an increased risk of instability and prosthetic dislocation following THA in patients with a history of alcohol misuse.[13,14] This increased risk may be related to increased association with liver disease, immunologic dysfunction, falls, adherence to precautions, and prosthetic joint infection.[15,16]

[a] Department of Orthopaedic Surgery, Tulane University School of Medicine, 1430 Tulane Avenue, New Orleans, LA 70112, USA; [b] Adult Reconstruction Hip/Knee, Department of Orthopaedic Surgery, Tulane University School of Medicine, 1430 Tulane Avenue, New Orleans, LA 70112, USA
* Corresponding author.
E-mail address: swilliam1@tulane.edu

Orthop Clin N Am 52 (2021) 191–200
https://doi.org/10.1016/j.ocl.2021.03.001

Higher body mass index (BMI) has been linked to increased risk of instability for patients with a BMI greater than 25,[17] BMI greater than 30,[18] and BMI greater than 35.[19] Similarly, Tohidi and colleagues[20] found increased risks of revision (relative risk [RR], 1.43; 95% CI, 0.96–2.13) and dislocation (RR, 2.38; 95% CI, 1.38–4.10) in men with BMI greater than 45. Higher BMI may lead to early instability because of increased risk of malpositioning of the implant during the index procedure.[21] However, the relationship between higher BMI and higher risk of instability or related mechanical complications has not been universally established,[22–24] and the efficacy of targeted weight loss programs before THA is unclear.[25] Furthermore, patients with higher BMI can obtain comparable clinical and functional outcomes following THA compared with patients with lower BMI.[26]

Nonmodifiable Patient Risk Factors

Many nonmodifiable risk factors for instability after THA have been established, including advanced age,[27,28] cognitive impairment,[29] and patient sex (Table 1). However, the current evidence for patient sex as a risk factor for THA instability and dislocation is mixed. Early studies suggested female sex was associated with a substantially higher risk of dislocation compared with men.[7,30] However, more recent studies have found no significant differences in rates of implant dislocation or instability-related revision procedures between men and women.[29,31] The higher incidence of instability in women may be more attributable to the smaller size of the femoral head implant[32,33] often used rather than an inherent anatomic predisposition.

Several comorbid conditions also predisposing patients to dislocation following THA include developmental dysplasia of the hip,[34] neuromuscular disorders,[35,36] and connective tissue diseases.[37,38] Strategies such as use of dual-mobility acetabular cups,[39] larger head size, and a direct anterior approach[40] have proved effective in reducing instability and dislocation in such high-risk patients. Prior hip surgery is also associated with increased risk of dislocation, including procedures such as fixation of intertrochanteric fractures via cephalomedullary nailing,[41] rotational acetabular osteotomy,[41] and hemiarthroplasty.[42]

Reduced spinopelvic mobility has recently garnered much attention in relation to THA instability. When a patient stands from a seated position, the degree of lordosis in the lumbar spine decreases, which causes the pelvis to tilt posteriorly and the sacrum and coccyx to rotate posteroinferiorly. This movement causes anteversion of the acetabular cup in response to femoral flexion.[43] In patients with degenerative disease or fusion of the lumbosacral spine, reduced spinopelvic mobility prevents the acetabulum from opening to the normal degree, which increases femur flexion, impingement of the anterior acetabulum, and risk of posterior prosthetic dislocation.[43–46] Prior studies show high rates of instability and prosthetic dislocation in patients with lumbar fusion and ankylosing spondylitis.[47,48]

Understanding the relationship between patients' unique pelvic dynamics and the risk of THA instability is paramount for accurate preoperative risk stratification and operative planning of implant positioning. Lum and colleagues[43] suggest routine measurement of the difference in sacral tilt (angle between a line parallel to the sacral end plate and a horizontal reference line) between the sitting and standing positions in all patients preoperatively, with corresponding recommendations for altered implant positioning. Lateral radiographs allow quick measurement of these angles, although recent research suggests radiographs in the flexed-seated or step-up positions better show a patient's range of spinopelvic motion.[49] However, surgeons may not be reliable in making these spinopelvic measurements accurately.[50]

Patients with reduced spinopelvic motion (ie, sacral tilt difference <10° between sitting and standing) are at an increased risk of implant dislocation with direction dependent on degree of mobility: patients with sacral tilt greater than 30° when standing have increased risk of anterior impingement and posterior dislocation, whereas fixed sacral tilt greater than 30° while sitting may cause posterior impingement and anterior dislocation.[43] In patients with prior lumbar spinal fusion, use of an anterior surgical approach and larger femoral head sizes can reduce rates of implant dislocation.[51,52] Such strategies would likely also benefit a broader group of patients undergoing THA, because most patients with a clinically stiff spine do not have a history of instrumented fusion.[53] However, generalized ranges of optimal cup anteversion and inclination remain unclear at a broad level.[54,55]

INTRAOPERATIVE RISK FACTORS
Approach

A primary surgical factor is the choice of approach to expose the femoroacetabular joint. Historically, the posterior approach has been associated with a higher incidence of dislocation compared with the anterolateral approach.[56] In

Table 1
Risk factors for instability after total hip arthroplasty and recommended interventions

Risk Factor	Intervention
Tobacco/alcohol abuse	• Preoperative cessation counseling
Advanced age	• Consideration of dual-mobility liner • Elevated liner
Obesity	• Weight loss programs
Neuromuscular and connective tissue disorders	• Dual-mobility liner • Direct anterior approach
Reduced spinopelvic mobility	• Standard preoperative imaging • Larger femoral head sizes ($\geq$32 mm) • Increased anteversion, inclination, and combined anteversion of implant for posterior approaches • Robotic-assisted implant design and positioning
Posterior approach	• Intraoperative repair of posterior capsule and local musculature • Consideration of elevated liner

1982, Woo and colleagues[7] reported a dislocation rate of 5.8% for patients undergoing a posterior approach compared with 2.3% in the anterolateral approach. However, over the past decades, multiple studies have shown dislocation rates of less than 1% while using a posterior approach when meticulous repair of the posterior capsule and musculature were performed.[57,58]

The direct anterior approach (DAA) has become more popular because of preservation of the posterior structures.[59] Compared with the posterolateral approach, surgeons performing the DAA achieved lower variance in both cup inclination and anteversion.[60,61] Numerous studies show the DAA provides increased dynamic hip stability and decreased dislocation after surgery, with large case series reporting dislocation rates of 0.60% to 0.96%.[62,63] In a series of 437 primary hips performed with a DAA, Matta and colleagues[64] documented a dislocation rate of 0.61%. Angerame and colleagues[65] reviewed 2431 DAA THAs and 4463 posterior THAs and reported a significantly lower rate of dislocation for the DAA (0.25%) compared with the posterior approach (0.49%). Using a large total joint registry consisting of more than 22,000 THAs, Sheth and colleagues[66] showed a significantly higher dislocation rate for the posterior

approach (1.4%) than the anterolateral approach (0.4%) and the DAA (0.8%).

A new technique described as a supercapsular percutaneously assisted (SuperPATH) approach has become widely popular because it promotes early mobilization and stability.[67] Major advantages of the SuperPATH approach include preservation of the external rotator musculature, the posterior hip capsule, and abductors, which provides increased stability and reduces incidence of posterior dislocation.[67] However, long-term outcome data for the SuperPATH approach are needed to determine its validity.

With improved closure techniques, surgeons have been able to reduce the incidence of dislocations when using a posterior approach; however, surgeons who use the DAA or anterolateral approach continue to achieve a lower incidence of dislocation.

Component Positioning
Accurate positioning of the femoral and acetabular components is paramount in constructing a dynamically stable THA. Orientation of the acetabular cup has often been regarded as the most critical for achieving dynamic stability because malpositioning of the cup is more common than the femoral component.[68] A safe zone for

component placement introduced by Lewinnek and colleagues[69] recommends placing the acetabular component in 40° ± 10° of abduction and 15° ± 10° of anteversion to minimize risk of dislocation because, outside of these ranges, the rate of dislocation increased from 1.5% to 6% while using a posterior approach. However, recent studies question the validity of the safe zone. In 2016, Abdel and colleagues[55] reported that 58% of patients with implant dislocation were within the safe zone parameters originally described by Lewinnek and colleagues.[69] Safe zones have not been well defined for DAA because the acute risk is higher for anterior dislocation.

For patients with deficient acetabular bone stock, it is difficult to achieve adequate bone coverage of the acetabular cup. Vertical placement of the cup has been proposed as a strategy to combat this challenge.[70] Initial studies accepted a maximum vertically displaced center of rotation of 35 mm for optimizing bone coverage while preventing substantial loss of range of motion.[71,72] In contrast, a more recent study reported that a vertically displaced center of rotation of greater than 23.9 mm resulted in a significantly increased risk of dislocation.[73]

IMPLANT CONFIGURATION
Femoral Head Size
Increasing the femoral head size provides 2 main advantages with regard to stability in THA. First, femoral heads with larger radii are seated deeper within the acetabular liner, resulting in an increased jump distance necessary to dislocate.[74–76] Although early studies failed to provide a correlation between head size and instability in THA, more recent studies show a significantly lower risk of dislocation with increased head size.[75,76] However, despite decreased dislocation risk, use of femoral head size greater than 32 mm carries an increased risk of polyethylene wear and trunnionosis by increasing the torsional forces on the trunnion, which may result in subsequent adverse local tissue reactions.[77]

Head to Neck Ratio
Increasing the head size or using a smaller diameter neck increases the head to neck ratio, allowing greater range of impingement-free motion.[78–80] Bader and colleagues[81] showed that a larger head to neck ratio leads to an increase in range of motion before impingement, range of motion before dislocation, and an increase in the resisting moment in subluxation. The investigators subsequently proposed that the head to neck ratio should be greater than 2:1 to optimize stability.[82] Increasing the femoral offset can also affect the

range of motion. In a cadaveric study, Matsushita and colleagues[83] reported that increasing the femoral offset to 4 mm and 8 mm led to 21.1° and 26.7° of improved flexion and 13.7° and 21.2° of improved rotation, respectively. In addition to increasing range of motion, an increased femoral offset adds tension to the surrounding soft tissues, particularly the abductor muscles, improving the stability of the prothesis.[84]

Acetabular Liner Profile
The morphology of the acetabular liner can also affect the stability of THA. A liner with an elevated rim of 15° placed in the posterior quadrant can provide increased stability by increasing the amount of internal rotation before subluxation by 8.9°.[85] Cobb and colleagues[86] compared neutral liners with 10° elevated rim liners in more than 5000 THAs and reported a significantly lower rate of dislocation in the elevated rim liners (2.19% vs 3.85%) at 2 years postoperatively. However, the added benefits of increased stability are offset by decreased extension and external rotation, and chronic impingement associated with these limitations can lead to increased polyethylene wear and component loosening over time.[68,86] Lateral offset liners can also be used in scenarios where reconstructed femoral offset is reduced or the acetabular component is medialized compared with the contralateral hip. In a series of 668 THAs performed through a posterior approach, a dislocation rate of 1.3% was reported and most of the dislocated hips had negative combined offset and abduction angles.[87]

Dual-mobility Implants
Dual-mobility implants offer surgeons an option for reducing dislocation risk by increasing the head to neck ratio and the arc of motion before impingement.[88] Various studies have reported a lower incidence of dislocation compared with fixed-bearing THA liners.[88] Rowan and colleagues[89] reported a dislocation ate of 0% (0 out of 136) for the dual-mobility cohort and 5.1% (7 out of 136) for the fixed-bearing cohort in a study of patients less than 55 years old. Although rare, with a reported incidence of 0.3% at 10 years, use of dual-mobility liners may result in a unique complication consisting of intraprosthetic dislocation, which almost always requires an open reduction and may decrease long-term survivorship.[90,91] Current literature suggests dual-mobility implants are an effective measure in reducing risk of instability; however, surgeons must weigh the clinical benefits against the addition of another bearing surface.

ROLE OF ROBOTICS/TECHNOLOGICAL ADVANCES IN REDUCING RATES OF INSTABILITY

Technology-assisted THA uses computer-assisted navigation and/or robotic assistance to increase surgeons' precision and accuracy in component positioning. From 2005 to 2014, use of technology-assisted THA increased from comprising 0.1% to 3.0% of all THAs being performed in the United States.[92]

ROBODOC (THINK Surgical, CA) was the first robotic-assisted system developed to aid surgeons with THA. Since 1994, more than 17,000 THAs have been performed worldwide with the assistance of ROBODOC despite not receiving US Food and Drug Administration (FDA) clearance in the United States until 2008.[93] In the first ROBODOC randomized controlled trial, 136 THAs performed between 1994 and 1995 compared ROBODOC-assisted THA with manual THA. Bargar and colleagues[94] reported the femoral component had a statistically better fit and position in the ROBODOC cohort by evaluation of postoperative radiographs and comparable Harris Hip Scores. In 2018, Bargar and colleagues[93] published the 14-year follow-up results of their single-surgeon randomized controlled trial, which failed to show a significant difference in outcomes between ROBODOC-assisted THA and manual THA. Additional studies since the landmark Bargar and colleagues[94] study have shown that ROBODOC-assisted THA can improve component positioning and reduce leg-length discrepancies compared with manual techniques.[95,96] In contrast, a prospective randomized control trial by Honl and colleagues[95] reported that the dislocation rate of 18% (11 out of 61) for the ROBODOC-assisted THAs was significantly higher than the 4% (3 out of 80) rate in the manual THA cohort. The investigators attributed the higher dislocation rate to intraoperative muscle damage caused by the robotic milling system. Despite the heterogenous results shown by ROBODOC studies, other robotic-assisted surgical systems have since emerged.

The MAKO robotic arm–assist system, which uses preoperative computed tomography (CT) scans and a robotic arm (MAKO; Stryker, NJ), received FDA approval in 2010 for THA, and its use continues to grow in popularity. Using the Lewinnek safe zone to define accuracy, Illgen and colleagues[97] reported that MAKO-assisted THAs achieved a 71% improvement in accuracy and a significantly lower dislocation rate (0% vs 3%; $P<.001$) at 2 years postoperatively in 100 robotic-assisted THAs compared with manual THA. Nawabi and colleagues[98] showed that MAKO robotic arm–assisted THA had 4 to 6 times greater accuracy with regard to version and inclination compared with manual THA. In a multicenter study, MAKO robotic arm–assisted THA's cup placement was within 5° of preoperative planned cup placement in 95% of procedures, showing the ability to assist surgeons with tailored patient-specific planning.[99] Kamara and colleagues[100] performed a retrospective review comparing 100 manual THAs, 100 fluoroscopic-assisted anterior THAs, and 100 robotic-assisted THAs and showed that component positioning was within the target zone in 76% of manual, 84% of fluoroscopic-assisted, and 97% of robotic-assisted procedures. The investigators also reported that the learning curve associated with robotic arm–assisted THAs is minimal and immediate improvement in precision of acetabular component position can be achieved. In addition, in 2018, a meta-analysis involving 522 robotic arm–assisted THAs and 994 manual THAs showed that the robotic cohort had more satisfactory cup placement, stem placement, and global offset compared with manual THA.[101]

Patients who are at an increased risk of instability preoperatively, such as those with reduced spinopelvic motion, can benefit from robotics because it assists surgeons in placing implant components in the optimal position per their unique anatomy. Snijders and colleagues[102] recently showed that the impact of sagittal pelvic dynamics on three-dimensional reorientation of the acetabular cup is specific to the unique initial acetabular cup orientation (ie, individual patients). Therefore, a movement away from recommendations based on broad categories and toward more individualized perioperative planning may be improved with the use of robotics by more accurately defining and understanding the dynamic spinopelvic mobility and impingement zones unique to each patient undergoing THA. With the use of robotics, a sitting and supine radiograph is combined with a CT scan to achieve optimal implant positioning and reduce impingement zones. Robotics also improves the ability to obtain accurate femoral offset calculations, calculate accurate combined anteversion, and restore leg length to a desired amount.[100,101,103]

SUMMARY

Instability is a major cause of failed primary THA and accounts for more than 22% of revisions. Anterior surgical approaches, larger femoral heads, high-offset stems, dual-mobility implants, and elevated/lipped liners can reduce the risk of instability postoperatively. Advances in robotic technology may improve understanding of spinopelvic mobility and aid in ideal component positioning through individualized surgical planning on dynamic three-dimensional models.

CLINICS CARE POINTS

- Larger femoral heads provide stability by increasing the head to neck ratio, providing greater range of motion and increased jump distance necessary for the head to displace. However, prosthetic heads greater than 32 mm can increase polyethylene wear and trunnionosis.

- A universal safe zone for acetabular cup placement has not yet been established, and surgeons must base placement on each patient's individualized anatomy and physiology.

- Robotic arm–assisted THA improves accuracy in implant placement and allows spinopelvic dynamic three-dimensional planning.

DISCLOSURE

The authors have nothing to disclose.

REFERENCES

1. Learmonth ID, Young C, Rorabeck C. The operation of the century: total hip replacement. Lancet 2007;370(9597):1508–19.

2. Bengtsson A, Donahue GS, Nemes S, et al. Consistency in patient-reported outcomes after total hip replacement. Acta Orthop 2017;88(5):484–9.

3. Wylde V, Blom AW, Whitehouse SL, et al. Patient-reported outcomes after total hip and knee arthroplasty: comparison of midterm results. J Arthroplasty 2009;24(2):210–6.

4. Berry DJ, Harmsen WS, Cabanela ME, et al. Twenty-five-year survivorship of two thousand consecutive primary Charnley total hip replacements: factors affecting survivorship of acetabular and femoral components. J Bone Joint Surg Am 2002;84(2):171–7.

5. Homesley HD, Minnich JM, Parvizi J, et al. Total hip arthroplasty revision: a decade of change. Am J Orthop (Belle Mead Nj) 2004;33(8):389–92.

6. Parvizi J, Kim KI, Goldberg G, et al. Recurrent instability after total hip arthroplasty: beware of subtle component malpositioning. Clin Orthop Relat Res 2006;447:60–5.

7. Woo RY, Morrey BF. Dislocations after total hip arthroplasty. J Bone Joint Surg Am 1982;64(9):1295–306.

8. Bozic KJ, Kurtz SM, Lau E, et al. The epidemiology of revision total hip arthroplasty in the United States. J Bone Joint Surg Am 2009;91(1):128–33.

9. Kurtz S, Ong K, Lau E, et al. Projections of primary and revision hip and knee arthroplasty in the United States from 2005 to 2030. J Bone Joint Surg Am 2007;89(4):780–5.

10. Pirruccio K, Premkumar A, Sheth NP. The burden of prosthetic hip dislocations in the United States is projected to significantly increase by 2035. Hip Int 2020. https://doi.org/10.1177/1120700020923619. 1120700020923619.

11. Lombardi AV Jr, Berend KR, Adams JB, et al. Smoking may be a harbinger of early failure with ultraporous metal acetabular reconstruction. Clin Orthop Relat Res 2013;471(2):486–97.

12. Chen Y, Guo Q, Pan X, et al. Smoking and impaired bone healing: will activation of cholinergic anti-inflammatory pathway be the bridge? Int Orthop 2011;35(9):1267–70.

13. Fini M, Giavaresi G, Salamanna F, et al. Harmful lifestyles on orthopedic implantation surgery: a descriptive review on alcohol and tobacco use. J Bone Miner Metab 2011;29(6):633–44.

14. Best MJ, Buller LT, Gosthe RG, et al. Alcohol misuse is an independent risk factor for poorer postoperative outcomes following primary total hip and total knee arthroplasty. J Arthroplasty 2015;30(8):1293–8.

15. Kong L, Cao J, Zhang Y, et al. Risk factors for periprosthetic joint infection following primary total hip or knee arthroplasty: a meta-analysis. Int Wound J 2017;14(3):529–36.

16. Lenguerrand E, Whitehouse MR, Beswick AD, et al. Risk factors associated with revision for prosthetic joint infection after hip replacement: a prospective observational cohort study. Lancet Infect Dis 2018;18(9):1004–14.

17. Sadr Azodi O, Adami J, Lindstrom D, et al. High body mass index is associated with increased risk of implant dislocation following primary total hip replacement: 2,106 patients followed for up to 8 years. Acta Orthop 2008;79(1):141–7.

18. Haverkamp D, Klinkenbijl MN, Somford MP, et al. Obesity in total hip arthroplasty–does it really matter? A meta-analysis. Acta Orthop 2011;82(4):417–22.

19. Wagner ER, Kamath AF, Fruth KM, et al. Effect of Body Mass Index on Complications and Reoperations After Total Hip Arthroplasty. J Bone Joint Surg Am 2016;98(3):169–79.

20. Tohidi M, Brogly SB, Lajkosz K, et al. Ten-year risk of complication and mortality after total hip arthroplasty in morbidly obese patients: a population study. Can J Surg 2019;62(6):442–9.

21. Callanan MC, Jarrett B, Bragdon CR, et al. The John Charnley Award: risk factors for cup malpositioning: quality improvement through a joint registry at a tertiary hospital. Clin Orthop Relat Res 2011;469(2):319–29.

22. Correa-Valderrama A, Stangl-Herrera W, Echeverry-Velez A, et al. Relationship between body mass index and complications during the first 45 days after primary total hip and knee replacement: a single-center study from South America. Clin Orthop Surg 2019;11(2):159–63.

23. Haynes J, Nam D, Barrack RL. Obesity in total hip arthroplasty: does it make a difference? Bone Joint J 2017;99-B(1 Supple A):31–6.

24. Hung CY, Chang CH, Lin YC, et al. Predictors for unfavorable early outcomes in elective total hip arthroplasty: does extreme body mass index matter? Biomed Res Int 2019;2019:4370382.

25. Lui M, Jones CA, Westby MD. Effect of nonsurgical, non-pharmacological weight loss interventions in patients who are obese prior to hip and knee arthroplasty surgery: a rapid review. Syst Rev 2015;4:121.

26. Li W, Ayers DC, Lewis CG, et al. Functional gain and pain relief after total joint replacement according to obesity status. J Bone Joint Surg Am 2017;99(14):1183–9.

27. Ezquerra-Herrando L, Seral-Garcia B, Quilez MP, et al. Instability of total hip replacement: A clinical study and determination of its risk factors. Rev Esp Cir Ortop Traumatol 2015;59(4):287–94.

28. Yang Q, Wang J, Xu Y, et al. Incidence and risk factors of in-hospital prosthesis-related complications following total hip arthroplasty: a retrospective Nationwide Inpatient Sample database study. Int Orthop 2020;44(11):2243–52.

29. Fessy MH, Putman S, Viste A, et al. What are the risk factors for dislocation in primary total hip arthroplasty? A multicenter case-control study of 128 unstable and 438 stable hips. Orthop Traumatol Surg Res 2017;103(5):663–8.

30. Ali Khan MA, Brakenbury PH, Reynolds IS. Dislocation following total hip replacement. J Bone Joint Surg Br 1981;63-B(2):214–8.

31. Inacio MC, Ake CF, Paxton EW, et al. Sex and risk of hip implant failure: assessing total hip arthroplasty outcomes in the United States. JAMA Intern Med 2013;173(6):435–41.

32. Bystrom S, Espehaug B, Furnes O, et al. Femoral head size is a risk factor for total hip luxation: a study of 42,987 primary hip arthroplasties from the Norwegian Arthroplasty Register. Acta Orthop Scand 2003;74(5):514–24.

33. Warschawski Y, Garceau SP, Joly DA, et al. The effect of femoral head size, neck length, and offset on dislocation rates of constrained acetabular liners. J Arthroplasty 2020;36(1):345–8.

34. Yetkin C, Yildirim T, Alpay Y, et al. Evaluation of dislocation risk factors with total hip arthroplasty in developmental hip dysplasia patients: a multivariate analysis. J Arthroplasty 2020;36(2):636–40.

35. Houdek MT, Watts CD, Wyles CC, et al. Total hip arthroplasty in patients with cerebral palsy: a cohort study matched to patients with osteoarthritis. J Bone Joint Surg Am 2017;99(6):488–93.

36. Murotani Y, Kuroda Y, Goto K, et al. Unexpected dislocation following accurate total hip arthroplasty caused by excessive hip joint laxity during myasthenic crisis: a case report. J Med Case Rep 2018;12(1):331.

37. Aziz KT, Best MJ, Skolasky RL, et al. Lupus and Perioperative Complications in Elective Primary Total Hip or Knee Arthroplasty. Clin Orthop Surg 2020;12(1):37–42.

38. Ravi B, Croxford R, Hollands S, et al. Increased risk of complications following total joint arthroplasty in patients with rheumatoid arthritis. Arthritis Rheumatol 2014;66(2):254–63.

39. Harwin SF, Mistry JB, Chughtai M, et al. Dual mobility acetabular cups in primary total hip arthroplasty in patients at high risk for dislocation. Surg Technol Int 2017;30:251–8.

40. Ochi H, Baba T, Homma Y, et al. Total hip arthroplasty via the direct anterior approach with a dual mobility cup for displaced femoral neck fracture in patients with a high risk of dislocation. SICOT J 2017;3:56.

41. Smith A, Denehy K, Ong KL, et al. Total hip arthroplasty following failed intertrochanteric hip fracture fixation treated with a cephalomedullary nail. Bone Joint J 2019;101-B(6_Supple_B):91–6.

42. Hernandez NM, Fruth KM, Larson DR, et al. Conversion of Hemiarthroplasty to THA carries an increased risk of reoperation compared with primary and revision THA. Clin Orthop Relat Res 2019;477(6):1392–9.

43. Lum ZC, Giordani M, Meehan JP. Total hip instability and the spinopelvic link. Curr Rev Musculoskelet Med 2020;13(4):425–34.

44. Ranawat CS, Ranawat AS, Lipman JD, et al. Effect of spinal deformity on pelvic orientation from standing to sitting position. J Arthroplasty 2016; 31(6):1222–7.

45. Buckland AJ, Vigdorchik J, Schwab FJ, et al. Acetabular anteversion changes due to spinal deformity correction: bridging the gap between hip and spine surgeons. J Bone Joint Surg Am 2015;97(23):1913–20.

46. Esposito CI, Miller TT, Kim HJ, et al. Does degenerative lumbar spine disease influence femoroacetabular flexion in patients undergoing total hip arthroplasty? Clin Orthop Relat Res 2016;474(8): 1788–97.

47. Buckland AJ, Puvanesarajah V, Vigdorchik J, et al. Dislocation of a primary total hip arthroplasty is more common in patients with a lumbar spinal fusion. Bone Joint J 2017;99-b(5):585–91.

48. Katakam A, Bedair HS, Melnic CM. Do all rigid and unbalanced spines present the same risk of dislocation after total hip arthroplasty? a comparison study between patients with ankylosing spondylitis and history of spinal fusion. J Arthroplasty 2020;35(12):3594.

49. Behery OA, Vasquez-Montes D, Cizmic Z, et al. Can flexed-seated and single-leg standing radiographs be useful in preoperative evaluation of lumbar mobility in total hip arthroplasty? J Arthroplasty 2020;35(8):2124–30.

50. Kleeman-Forsthuber LT, Elkins JM, Miner TM, et al. Reliability of spinopelvic measurements that may influence the cup position in total hip arthroplasty. J Arthroplasty 2020;35(12):3758–64.

51. Mononen H, Sund R, Halme J, et al. Following total hip arthroplasty: femoral head component diameter of 32 mm or larger is associated with lower risk of dislocation in patients with a prior lumbar fusion. Bone Joint J 2020;102-B(8):1003–9.

52. Kahn TL, Kellam PJ, Anderson LA, et al. Can dislocation rates be decreased using the anterior approach in patients with lumbar spondylosis or lumbar instrumented fusion? J Arthroplasty 2021; 36(1):217–21.

53. Vigdorchik JM, Sharma AK, Dennis DA, et al. The majority of total hip arthroplasty patients with a stiff spine do not have an instrumented fusion. J Arthroplasty 2020;35(6S):S252–4.

54. Seagrave KG, Troelsen A, Malchau H, et al. Acetabular cup position and risk of dislocation in primary total hip arthroplasty. Acta Orthop 2017; 88(1):10–7.

55. Abdel MP, von Roth P, Jennings MT, et al. What safe zone? the vast majority of dislocated THAs are within the lewinnek safe zone for acetabular component position. Clin Orthop Relat Res 2016;474(2):386–91.

56. Masonis JL, Bourne RB. Surgical approach, abductor function, and total hip arthroplasty dislocation. Clin Orthop Relat Res 2002;(405): 46–53.

57. Goldstein WM, Gleason TF, Kopplin M, et al. Prevalence of dislocation after total hip arthroplasty through a posterolateral approach with partial capsulotomy and capsulorrhaphy. J Bone Joint Surg Am 2001;83-A Suppl 2(Pt 1):2–7.

58. White RE Jr, Forness TJ, Allman JK, et al. Effect of posterior capsular repair on early dislocation in primary total hip replacement. Clin Orthop Relat Res 2001;(393):163–7.

59. Barrett WP, Turner SE, Leopold JP. Prospective randomized study of direct anterior vs postero-

lateral approach for total hip arthroplasty. J Arthroplasty 2013;28(9):1634–8.

60. Zhao HY, Kang PD, Xia YY, et al. Comparison of early functional recovery after total hip arthroplasty using a direct anterior or posterolateral approach: a randomized controlled trial. J Arthroplasty 2017;32(11):3421–8.

61. Fransen B, Hoozemans M, Vos S. Direct anterior approach versus posterolateral approach in total hip arthroplasty : one surgeon, two approaches. Acta Orthop Belg 2016;82(2):240–8.

62. Anterior Total Hip Arthroplasty Collaborative Investigators, Bhandari M, Matta JM, et al. Outcomes following the single-incision anterior approach to total hip arthroplasty: a multicenter observational study. Orthop Clin North Am 2009; 40(3):329–42.

63. Siguier T, Siguier M, Brumpt B. Mini-incision anterior approach does not increase dislocation rate: a study of 1037 total hip replacements. Clin Orthop Relat Res 2004;(426):164–73.

64. Matta JM, Shahrdar C, Ferguson T. Single-incision anterior approach for total hip arthroplasty on an orthopaedic table. Clin Orthop Relat Res 2005; 441:115–24.

65. Angerame MR, Fehring TK, Masonis JL, et al. Early failure of primary total hip arthroplasty: is surgical approach a risk factor? J Arthroplasty 2018;33(6): 1780–5.

66. Sheth D, Cafri G, Inacio MC, et al. Anterior and anterolateral approaches for THA are associated with lower dislocation risk without higher revision risk. Clin Orthop Relat Res 2015;473(11):3401–8.

67. Chow J. SuperPath: The direct superior portal-assisted total hip approach. JBJS Essent Surg Tech 2017;7(3):e23.

68. Sanchez-Sotelo J, Berry DJ. Epidemiology of instability after total hip replacement. Orthop Clin North Am 2001;32(4):543–52, vii.

69. Lewinnek GE, Lewis JL, Tarr R, et al. Dislocations after total hip-replacement arthroplasties. J Bone Joint Surg Am 1978;60(2):217–20.

70. Russotti GM, Harris WH. Proximal placement of the acetabular component in total hip arthroplasty. A long-term follow-up study. J Bone Joint Surg Am 1991;73(4):587–92.

71. Doehring TC, Rubash HE, Shelley FJ, et al. Effect of superior and superolateral relocations of the hip center on hip joint forces. An experimental and analytical analysis. J Arthroplasty 1996;11(6): 693–703.

72. Komiyama K, Nakashima Y, Hirata M, et al. Does high hip center decrease range of motion in total hip arthroplasty? a computer simulation study. J Arthroplasty 2016;31(10):2342–7.

73. Komiyama K, Fukushi JI, Motomura G, et al. Does high hip centre affect dislocation after total hip

arthroplasty for developmental dysplasia of the hip? Int Orthop 2019;43(9):2057–63.

74. Soong M, Rubash HE, Macaulay W. Dislocation after total hip arthroplasty. J Am Acad Orthop Surg 2004;12(5):314–21.

75. Berry DJ, von Knoch M, Schleck CD, et al. Effect of femoral head diameter and operative approach on risk of dislocation after primary total hip arthroplasty. J Bone Joint Surg Am 2005; 87(11):2456–63.

76. Dudda M, Gueleryuez A, Gautier E, et al. Risk factors for early dislocation after total hip arthroplasty: a matched case-control study. J Orthop Surg (Hong Kong) 2010;18(2):179–83.

77. Lachiewicz PF, Soileau ES, Martell JM. Wear and Osteolysis of Highly Crosslinked Polyethylene at 10 to 14 Years: The Effect of Femoral Head Size. Clin Orthop Relat Res 2016;474(2):365–71.

78. Amstutz HC, Lodwig RM, Schurman DJ, et al. Range of motion studies for total hip replacements. A comparative study with a new experimental apparatus. Clin Orthop Relat Res 1975; 111:124–30.

79. Krushell RJ, Burke DW, Harris WH. Range of motion in contemporary total hip arthroplasty. The impact of modular head-neck components. J Arthroplasty 1991;6(2):97–101.

80. Bunn A, Colwell CW Jr, D'Lima DD. Effect of head diameter on passive and active dynamic hip dislocation. J Orthop Res 2014;32(11):1525–31.

81. Bader R, Steinhauser E, Gradinger R, et al. [Computer-based motion simulation of total hip prostheses with ceramic-on-ceramic wear couple. Analysis of implant design and orientation as influence parameters]. Z Orthop Ihre Grenzgeb 2002;140(3):310–6.

82. Bader R, Scholz R, Steinhauser E, et al. The influence of head and neck geometry on stability of total hip replacement: a mechanical test study. Acta Orthop Scand 2004;75(4):415–21.

83. Matsushita A, Nakashima Y, Jingushi S, et al. Effects of the femoral offset and the head size on the safe range of motion in total hip arthroplasty. J Arthroplasty 2009;24(4):646–51.

84. Girard J, Lavigne M, Vendittoli PA, et al. Biomechanical reconstruction of the hip: a randomised study comparing total hip resurfacing and total hip arthroplasty. J Bone Joint Surg Br 2006;88(6): 721–6.

85. Sultan PG, Tan V, Lai M, et al. Independent contribution of elevated-rim acetabular liner and femoral head size to the stability of total hip implants. J Arthroplasty 2002;17(3):289–92.

86. Cobb TK, Morrey BF, Ilstrup DM. The elevated-rim acetabular liner in total hip arthroplasty: relationship to postoperative dislocation. J Bone Joint Surg Am 1996;78(1):80–6.

87. Robinson M, Bornstein L, Mennear B, et al. Effect of restoration of combined offset on stability of large head THA. Hip Int 2012;22(3):248–53.

88. Scott TP, Weitzler L, Salvatore A, et al. A retrieval analysis of impingement in dual-mobility liners. J Arthroplasty 2018;33(8):2660–5.

89. Rowan FE, Salvatore AJ, Lange JK, et al. Dual-mobility vs fixed-bearing total hip arthroplasty in patients under 55 years of age: a single-institution, matched-cohort analysis. J Arthroplasty 2017; 32(10):3076–81.

90. Philippot R, Boyer B, Farizon F. Intraprosthetic dislocation: a specific complication of the dual-mobility system. Clin Orthop Relat Res 2013; 471(3):965–70.

91. Massin P, Orain V, Philippot R, et al. Fixation failures of dual mobility cups: a mid-term study of 2601 hip replacements. Clin Orthop Relat Res 2012;470(7):1932–40.

92. Hsiue PP, Chen CJ, Villalpando C, et al. Trends and patient factors associated with technology-assisted total hip arthroplasty in the United States from 2005 to 2014. Arthroplast Today 2020;6(1): 112–117 e111.

93. Bargar WL, Parise CA, Hankins A, et al. Fourteen year follow-up of randomized clinical trials of active robotic-assisted total hip arthroplasty. J Arthroplasty 2018;33(3):810–4.

94. Bargar WL, Bauer A, Borner M. Primary and revision total hip replacement using the Robodoc system. Clin Orthop Relat Res 1998;(354):82–91.

95. Honl M, Dierk O, Gauck C, et al. Comparison of robotic-assisted and manual implantation of a primary total hip replacement. A prospective study. J Bone Joint Surg Am 2003;85(8):1470–8.

96. Nakamura N, Sugano N, Nishii T, et al. A comparison between robotic-assisted and manual implantation of cementless total hip arthroplasty. Clin Orthop Relat Res 2010;468(4):1072–81.

97. Illgen RLN, Bukowski BR, Abiola R, et al. Robotic-assisted total hip arthroplasty: outcomes at minimum two-year follow-up. Surg Technol Int 2017; 30:365–72.

98. Nawabi DH, Conditt MA, Ranawat AS, et al. Haptically guided robotic technology in total hip arthroplasty: a cadaveric investigation. Proc Inst Mech Eng H 2013;227(3):302–9.

99. Elson L, Dounchis J, Illgen R, et al. Precision of acetabular cup placement in robotic integrated total hip arthroplasty. Hip Int 2015;25(6):531–6.

100. Kamara E, Robinson J, Bas MA, et al. Adoption of robotic vs fluoroscopic guidance in total hip arthroplasty: is acetabular positioning improved in the learning curve? J Arthroplasty 2017;32(1): 125–30.

101. Chen X, Xiong J, Wang P, et al. Robotic-assisted compared with conventional total hip

arthroplasty: systematic review and meta-analysis. Postgrad Med J 2018;94(1112):335–41.

102. Snijders TE, Schlosser TPC, van Stralen M, et al. The effect of postural pelvic dynamics on the three-dimensional orientation of the acetabular cup in THA Is Patient Specific. Clin Orthop Relat Res 2020;479(3):561–71.

103. Perets I, Mu BH, Mont MA, et al. Current topics in robotic-assisted total hip arthroplasty: a review. Hip Int 2020;30(2):118–24.

Blood Management in Outpatient Total Hip Arthroplasty

Samuel Gray McClatchy, MD*, Joseph T. Cline, MD,
Carson M. Rider, MD, Zachary K. Pharr, MD,
William M. Mihalko, MD, PhD, Patrick C. Toy, MD

KEYWORDS

- Outpatient total hip arthroplasty • Blood loss management • Protocol • Safety

---

KEY POINTS

- Blood loss requiring a blood transfusion has been cited as the leading complication following outpatient arthroplasty in the Medicare population.
- As outpatient arthroplasty becomes more common, there is an increased importance of blood management to prevent the need for blood transfusions.
- A blood management protocol that includes presurgical hematocrit of greater than 36%, administration of tranexamic acid, prophylactic introduction of albumin, hypotensive epidural anesthesia, monopolar electrocautery, and bipolar sealer can create a standardized and reproducible pathway that can increase the safety of outpatient hip arthroplasty.

INTRODUCTION

Over the past several years there has been a shift from inpatient hospital-based arthroplasty to outpatient ambulatory surgery center–based arthroplasty, with expectations that by the year 2026 more than half of all primary hip arthroplasties will be performed as outpatient procedure.[1,2] The cause for this shift is multifactorial. Economic benefits and the increased importance of cost savings and value-based care are largely responsible, as are improvements in pain management and recovery protocols and patients' desire to recover in the comfort of their own home.[3–6] As discharge from the ambulatory surgery center to home (DASH) arthroplasty increases, so does the importance of demonstrating safety and preventing potential complications.[7]

Greenky and colleagues reported that the leading complication following outpatient arthroplasty in the Medicare population was blood loss requiring a blood transfusion.[8] The safety of arthroplasty in an ambulatory surgery center has been questioned because of blood loss and the possible need for blood transfusions postoperatively, as these cannot be performed outside of the hospital setting. Blood loss following a primary total hip arthroplasty can be significant, and drops in hematocrit have been reported as −4.9 ± 3.2 on the day of surgery and −8.9 ± 4.7 on the first postoperative day.[9] As DASH arthroplasty becomes more common, there is an increased importance of blood management to prevent the need for blood transfusions.

Given the limitations of isolated ambulatory surgery centers, attention to blood loss and prevention of blood transfusions are essential. Multimodal pain management protocols and patient selection pathways have been shown to be critical for successful outpatient surgery[10,11]; however, to our knowledge, there have been no studies to date regarding blood management protocols for arthroplasty in the outpatient setting. We present results regarding blood loss

---

Department of Orthopaedic Surgery and Biomedical Engineering, University of Tennessee-Campbell Clinic, Memphis, TN, USA
* Corresponding author. 1211 Union Avenue, Suite 510, Memphis, TN 38104.
E-mail address: sgmcclatchy@gmail.com

Orthop Clin N Am 52 (2021) 201–208
https://doi.org/10.1016/j.ocl.2021.03.004
0030-5898/21/© 2021 Elsevier Inc. All rights reserved.

and transfusion rates from a single surgeon performing DASH outpatient arthroplasty over a 5-year period, specifically looking at the effect of bipolar sealer on blood loss and operative time, and propose a standardized protocol for blood loss management to reduce the need for blood transfusions.

METHODS

After Institutional Review Board approval, the records of all outpatient hip arthroplasties performed by a single surgeon over a 5-year period from 2013 to 2018 were retrospectively reviewed. Patients were excluded if the procedures were not performed at a stand-alone ambulatory surgery center.

All total hip arthroplasties were performed via the direct anterior approach. Monopolar electrocautery (Bovie, Symmetry Surgical, Antioch, TN, USA) was used intraoperatively in all cases, and bipolar sealer (Aquamantys, Minneapolis, MN, USA) was adopted after clinical benefit was seen from its use in inpatient arthroplasty. Tranexamic acid was given as 2 doses. For the preoperative dose, if intravenous, 1 g of tranexamic acid was administered within 1 hour before incision or 1950 mg (3 tablets of 650 mg) approximately 2 hours before incision if oral. For patients who initially received an intravenous dose, a second gram of tranexamic acid was given intravenously at the beginning of wound closure. There were no exclusions to the use of tranexamic acid. Albumin was provided as 500 mL of 5% human albumin, and hypotensive epidural anesthesia was used by the anesthesia team when possible, with a target mean arterial pressure of 60 mm Hg.

Data for all patients were analyzed for blood loss, hematocrit, comorbidities, patient demographics, and blood loss–related complications. Blood loss–related complications were defined as blood transfusions, symptomatic hypotension, or syncope. Statistical analysis consisted of univariate t-tests and analysis of variance comparing estimated blood loss with bipolar sealer use as well as with our variables of interest. A regression analysis was then performed on the variables that showed statistical significance or association to control for patient demographics and confounders.

RESULTS

The cohort consisted of 234 men (57.5%) and 173 women (42.5%), with a mean age of 55.8 years. The estimated blood loss ranged from 20 mL to 2000 mL, with a mean blood loss of 362.7 mL. The average preoperative hematocrit was 42.4 ± 4.1 and postoperative hematocrit was 35.0 ± 4.7. Full patient demographics are shown in Table 1.

A single patient (<0.01%) required transfer to an inpatient hospital facility for a blood transfusion, and 6 patients (0.01%) had syncopal episodes postoperatively. The patient with symptomatic postoperative anemia (hematocrit 25.9%) received a transfusion and was discharged uneventfully the following day. The 6 patients with syncopal episodes were provided intravenous fluids, and all were successfully discharged home the same day as surgery.

Comparing the estimated blood loss with and without bipolar sealer use showed a significant decrease with bipolar sealer use (431.1 mL vs 351.1 mL, $P<.01$); however, once a regression analysis was performed, this was no longer significant ($P>.05$). Patient demographics were broken down by bipolar sealer use (Table 2). Looking at operative times when using the bipolar sealer, there was a statistically significant decrease in surgery duration (80.4 ± 18.7 min vs 58.9 ± 11.5 min, $P<.01$).

In this study, 368 patients (90.4%) had hypotensive epidural anesthesia. Comparing the blood loss between spinal and general anesthesia, there was a statistically significant decrease in the estimated blood loss when spinal anesthesia was used (274.3 ± 209.1 vs 386.6 ± 229.8, $P<.01$); however, when controlling for confounders, this was not statistically significant.

DISCUSSION

Blood loss–related complications in this study were few. In total there were 7 incidences, with one patient requiring transfer to an inpatient hospital facility for blood transfusion. We hypothesized that this one transfusion could be due to many different factors. At the start of surgery, the patient had a preoperative hematocrit of 43.3% and had a significant blood loss (2000 mL) intraoperatively. Compared with the other patients, this single patient experienced the greatest blood loss by greater than 900 mL, which was found to be due to an undiagnosed blood dyscrasia. This patient also was early in the series (ninth), which may indicate a learning curve contributing to the complication. In addition, a bipolar sealer was not used in this patient's case. After bipolar sealer use was adopted for more thorough hemostasis, no blood transfusions were required.

The use of a bipolar sealer was not standardized in our study. Initially, only monopolar cautery was used (56 patients). After observing the clinical

Table 1 Patient demographics	
	THA (N = 407)
Gender	
Female	173 (42.5%)
Male	234 (57.5%)
Race	
White	330 (81.1%)
Black	65 (16.0%)
Other	12 (2.9%)
Age at surgery (y)	
Mean (SD)	55.8 (8.20)
Median [Min, Max]	57.2 [22.3, 72.9]
BMI (kg/m^2)	
Mean (SD)	30.0 (4.94)
Median [Min, Max]	29.9 [18.3, 52.9]
Pre-op HCT (%)	
Mean (SD)	42.4 (4.06)
Median [Min, Max]	42.3 [29.6, 54.0]
Post-op HCT (%)	
Mean (SD)	35.0 (4.67)
Median [Min, Max]	35.0 [23.0, 47.0]
EBL (mL)	
Mean (SD)	362 (209)
Median [Min, Max]	300 [20.0, 2000]
Surgery time (h)	
Mean (SD)	1.03 (0.244)
Median [Min, Max]	1.00 [0.483, 2.28]
ASA Score	
1	32 (7.9%)
2	277 (68.1%)
3	98 (24.1%)
Comorbidities	
Heart disease	36 (8.8%)
Chronic obstructive pulmonary disease	7 (1.7%)
Hypertension	205 (50.4%)
Diabetes	30 (7.4%)
Cerebrovascular accident	2 (0.5%)
DVT	9 (2.2%)
Tobacco use	29 (7.1%)
Anesthesia Type	
Spinal	368 (90.4%)
General	39 (9.6%)

(continued on next page)

	THA (N = 407)
Bipolar sealer use	
No	56 (13.8%)
Yes	351 (86.2%)
Postop Complications	
None	400 (98.3%)
Syncope	6 (1.5%)
Blood transfusion	1 (0.2%)

Abbreviations: ASA, American Society of Anesthesiologists; DVT, deep vein thrombosis; SD, standard deviation; THA, Total hip arthroplasty.

benefit of the bipolar sealer in hip arthroplasties in the hospital setting, the instrument was adopted for regular use with outpatient hip arthroplasties (351 patients). As a result, a comparison of the estimated blood loss with and without bipolar sealer was possible, and a significant decrease in estimated blood loss was found when bipolar sealer was used (univariate analysis, 431.1 mL vs 351.1 mL, $P<.01$). When we controlled for other demographics, however, this difference was no longer significant. Despite the lack of support for a significant decrease in estimated blood loss, there was a statistically significant decrease in surgery duration when using the bipolar sealer (80.4 ± 18.7 min vs 58.9 ± 11.5 min, $P<.01$), which we believe is due to time saved achieving hemostasis. The literature on bipolar sealer use is mixed. Although some studies have shown that bipolar sealer use is associated with decreased risk of blood transfusions and decreased length of stay,[12–14] some suggest a limited benefit of bipolar sealer on blood loss.[15,16] As the importance of value-based care increases, careful consideration of the cost and benefit of each instrument and implant is needed. At our ambulatory surgery center, one bipolar sealer handpiece costs $512.41, and each monopolar electrocautery with grounding pad costs $6.33. This cost difference is significant but may be worthwhile based on the benefit it provides. Although our results on the effect of bipolar sealers on estimated blood loss are inconclusive, they do suggest that the hemostatic device may significantly shorten operative times. Given these results, we believe it can be a useful adjunct; however, additional studies are needed.

As hip arthroplasty progresses from the inpatient to outpatient setting, it is critical to maintain patient safety and quality of care. Lovecchio and colleagues noted a need for pathways that include blood management protocols to minimize complications with outpatient arthroplasty.[17] Based on our series of outpatient total hip arthroplasties, we propose a standardized protocol for blood loss management in outpatient arthroplasty consisting of a presurgical hematocrit of greater than 36%, administration of tranexamic acid, prophylactic introduction of albumin, hypotensive epidural anesthesia, monopolar electrocautery, and bipolar sealer. This protocol uses techniques that alone are not novel but together create a standardized and reproducible pathway that has resulted in safe outpatient hip arthroplasty in a single ambulatory surgery center.

The antifibrinolytic drug tranexamic acid has been widely adopted among arthroplasty surgeons to decrease operative blood loss.[18] Tranexamic acid is a synthetic amino acid that functions as a clot stabilizer by competitively inhibiting the activation of plasminogen and degradation of the fibrin clot.[18,19] Tranexamic acid has consistently demonstrated its ability to decrease intraoperative blood loss and the need for blood transfusions postoperatively.[18,20,21] We believe tranexamic acid use to be critical to safely performing arthroplasty in the outpatient setting. All arthroplasty patients received systemic tranexamic acid without exclusions. Initially tranexamic acid was given only intravenously, but primarily oral administration was adopted because studies have shown equivalent efficacy of oral formulations at reducing blood loss at a fraction of the cost.[22–24] For optimal effect, oral tranexamic acid needs to be given 2 hours before incision versus within 1 hour with intravenous administration, therefore some patients were unable to receive oral dosing due to time constraints.[25]

Several studies have indicated that preoperative hematocrit or hemoglobin is an independent risk factor for blood transfusion following hip

Table 2
Comparison of patient demographics divided by bipolar sealer usage

	No Bipolar Sealer (N = 56)	Bipolar Sealer (N = 351)	Overall (N = 407)
Gender			
Female	21 (37.5%)	152 (43.3%)	173 (42.5%)
Male	35 (62.5%)	199 (56.7%)	234 (57.5%)
Race			
White	47 (83.9%)	283 (80.6%)	330 (81.1%)
Black	5 (8.9%)	60 (17.1%)	65 (16.0%)
Other	4 (7.1%)	8 (2.3%)	12 (2.9%)
Age at surgery (y)			
Mean (SD)	54.4 (8.37)	56.0 (8.16)	55.8 (8.20)
Median [Min, Max]	56.1 [27.7, 69.0]	57.3 [22.3, 72.9]	57.2 [22.3, 72.9]
BMI			
Mean (SD)	29.2 (4.04)	30.2 (5.06)	30.0 (4.94)
Median [Min, Max]	29.5 [19.6, 37.2]	30.0 [18.3, 52.9]	29.9 [18.3, 52.9]
Pre-op HCT (%)			
Mean (SD)	33.8 (4.33)	42.2 (4.02)	42.4 (4.06)
Median [Min, Max]	33.0 [25.9, 40.7]	42.4 [30.4, 49.3]	42.3 [29.6, 54.0]
Post-op HCT (%)			
Mean (SD)	35.2 (4.72)	42.4 (4.07)	35.0 (4.68)
Median [Min, Max]	35.0 [47.0, 23.0]	42.2 [29.6, 54.0]	35.0 [23.0, 47.0]
EBL (mL)			
Mean (SD)	431 (272)	351 (196)	362 (209)
Median [Min, Max]	350 [100, 2000]	300 [20.0, 1100]	300 [20.0, 2000]
Surgery time (h)			
Mean (SD)	1.34 (0.311)	0.981 (0.191)	1.03 (0.244)
Median [Min, Max]	1.33 [0.800, 2.28]	0.967 [0.483, 2.00]	1.00 [0.483, 2.28]
ASA Score			
1	4 (7.1%)	28 (8.0%)	32 (7.9%)
2	46 (82.1%)	231 (65.8%)	277 (68.1%)
3	6 (10.7%)	92 (26.2%)	98 (24.1%)
Comorbidities			
Heart disease	3 (5.4%)	33 (9.4%)	36 (8.8%)
Chronic obstructive pulmonary disease	1 (1.8%)	6 (1.7%)	7 (1.7%)
Hypertension	22 (39.3%)	183 (52.1%)	205 (50.4%)
Diabetes	4 (7.1%)	26 (7.4%)	30 (7.4%)
Cerebrovascular accident	0 (0%)	2 (0.6%)	2 (0.5%)
DVT	1 (1.8%)	8 (2.3%)	9 (2.2%)
Tobacco	4 (7.1%)	25 (7.1%)	29 (7.1%)

(continued on next page)

	No Bipolar Sealer (N = 56)	Bipolar Sealer (N = 351)	Overall (N = 407)
Anesthesia Type			
Spinal	51 (91.1%)	317 (90.3%)	368 (90.4%)
General	5 (8.9%)	34 (9.7%)	39 (9.6%)
Postop Complications			
None	53 (94.6%)	347 (98.9%)	400 (98.2%)
Syncope	2 (3.6%)	4 (1.1%)	6 (1.5%)
Blood transfusion	1 (1.8%)	0 (0%)	1 (0.2%)

Abbreviations: ASA, American Society of Anesthesiologists; BMI, body mass index; DVT, deep vein thrombosis; EBL, estimated blood loss; HCT, hematocrit; SD, standard deviation.

arthroplasty.[26,27] Yeh and colleagues[28] suggested hemoglobin cut-off values of 12.1 g/dL for patients younger than 70 years and 12.4 g/dL for patients older than 70 years and undergoing total joint arthroplasty.[27] Our protocol adopted a preoperative hematocrit cut-off of 36% for patients planning to have outpatient arthroplasty. Patients found to be anemic should be delayed at the operative surgeon's discretion until appropriate evaluation and correction can be completed.

Hypotensive epidural anesthesia is an additional measure that can decrease intraoperative blood loss and the risk of blood transfusions.[29–31] Although this technique is not appropriate for all patients, we have adopted hypotensive epidural anesthesia as our preferred method, with greater than 90% of arthroplasties in our study performed under spinal anesthesia. The primary reason patients did not receive epidural anesthesia was posterior spinal anatomy that precluded epidural access. In addition, prophylactic 5% human albumin was given along with crystalloid to mitigate the effect of blood loss as well as the lability of blood pressure associated with the epidural anesthesia. The use of colloids intraoperatively helps to maintain osmotic pressure in the intravascular space and support blood pressure.[32]

Outpatient joint arthroplasty can be successfully completed using carefully selected blood and pain management protocols. There are certainly other potential variables that have to considered. Some of those are related to the patient or facility itself, but the experience and expertise of the surgeon performing the joint arthroplasty is one factor often underemphasized. In addition to implementing a blood management protocol, it is recommended that the treating surgeon perform successful outpatient joint replacement in the hospital before scheduling cases in an ambulatory center.

This study is not without limitations. It carries the inherent bias of a case series with retrospective data collection. Also, estimated blood loss was used in this study for surgical blood loss, but this is not as objective as comparing preoperative with postoperative hematocrit levels. In our study, we were unable to make this comparison because postoperative hematocrit was not routinely collected and was reported in only 161 (39.6%) of 407 patients. In addition, the proposed standardized protocol was not implemented for all patients in this cohort and was adjusted after earlier outpatient arthroplasty cases to improve blood management and patient outcomes.

SUMMARY

Although blood transfusions make up only a small percentage of the overall complications of outpatient total joint arthroplasty, they are a costly complication. Despite the risks, outpatient total joints can be performed safely with a low risk of transfusion due to blood loss. Bipolar sealer is a useful instrument that may shorten operative times; its effect on reducing blood loss remains to be seen. The proposed protocol for managing blood loss may help lower the risk of transfusion for other surgeons participating in DASH arthroplasty.

CLINICS CARE POINTS

- Use of a bipolar sealer can significantly decrease surgery duration, resulting in less blood loss.
- Hypotensive epidural anesthesia also can decrease blood loss.

- In patients found to be anemic (hematocrit level less than 36%) surgery should be delayed at the operative surgeon's discretion until appropriate evaluation and correction can be completed.
- For optimal effect, oral tranexamic acid needs to be given 2 hours before incision versus within 1 hour with intravenous administration.

DISCLOSURE

The authors have nothing to disclose.

REFERENCES

1. DeCook CA. Outpatient joint arthroplasty: transitioning to the ambulatory surgery center. J Arthroplasty 2019;34(7):S48–50.
2. Berger RA, Cross MB, Sanders S. Outpatient hip and knee replacement: the experience from the first 15 years. Instr Course Lect 2016;65:547–51.
3. Aynardi M, Post Z, Ong A, et al. Outpatient surgery as a means of cost reduction in total hip arthroplasty: a case-control study. HSS J 2014;10(3):252–5.
4. Bertin KC. Minimally invasive outpatient total hip arthroplasty: a financial analysis. Clin Orthop Relat Res 2005;435:154–63.
5. Gogineni HC, Gray CF, Prieto HA, et al. Transition to outpatient total hip and knee arthroplasty: experience at an academic tertiary care center. Arthroplast Today 2019;5(1):100–5.
6. Kim S, Losina E, Solomon DH, et al. Effectiveness of clinical pathways for total knee and total hip arthroplasty: literature review. J Arthroplasty 2003;18(1):69–74.
7. McClatchy SG, Rider CM, Mihalko WM, et al. Defining outpatient hip and knee arthroplasties: a systematic review. J Am Acad Orthop Surg 2020. https://doi.org/10.5435/JAAOS-D-19-00636.
8. Greenky MR, Wang W, Ponzio DY, et al. Total hip arthroplasty and the Medicare Inpatient-Only List: an analysis of complications in Medicare-aged Patients undergoing outpatient surgery. J Arthroplasty 2019;34(6):1250–4.
9. Zhou Q, Zhou Y, Wu H, et al. Changes of hemoglobin and hematocrit in elderly patients receiving lower joint arthroplasty without allogeneic blood transfusion. Chin Med J 2015;128(1):75–8.
10. Hamilton WG. Protocol development for outpatient total joint arthroplasty. J Arthroplasty 2019;34(7):S46–7.
11. Toy PC, Fournier MN, Throckmorton TW, et al. Low rates of adverse events following ambulatory outpatient total hip arthroplasty at a free-standing surgery center. J Arthroplasty 2018;33(1):46–50.
12. Suarez JC, Slotkin EM, Szubski CR, et al. Prospective, randomized trial to evaluate efficacy of a bipolar sealer in direct anterior approach total hip arthroplasty. J Arthroplasty 2015;30(11):1953–8.
13. Ackerman SJ, Tapia CI, Baik R, et al. Use of a bipolar sealer in total hip arthroplasty: medical resource use and costs using a hospital administrative database. Orthopedics 2014;37(5):e472–81.
14. Min J-K, Zhang Q-H, Li H-D, et al. The efficacy of bipolar sealer on blood loss in primary total hip arthroplasty: a meta-analysis. Medicine (Baltimore) 2016;95(19):e3435.
15. Dabash S, Barksdale LC, McNamara CA, et al. Blood loss reduction with tranexamic acid and a bipolar sealer in direct anterior total hip arthroplasty. Am J Orthop 2018;47(5). https://doi.org/10.12788/ajo.2018.0032.
16. Huang Z, Ma J, Shen B, et al. Use of a bipolar blood-sealing system during total joint arthroplasty. Orthopedics 2015;38(12):757–63.
17. Lovecchio F, Alvi H, Sahota S, et al. Is outpatient arthroplasty as safe as fast-track inpatient arthroplasty? A propensity score matched analysis. J Arthroplasty 2016;31(9):197–201.
18. Fillingham YA, Ramkumar DB, Jevsevar DS, et al. The efficacy of tranexamic acid in total hip arthroplasty: a network meta-analysis. J Arthroplasty 2018;33(10):3083–9.e4.
19. Fillingham YA, Ramkumar DB, Jevsevar DS, et al. The safety of tranexamic acid in total joint arthroplasty: a direct meta-analysis. J Arthroplasty 2018;33(10):3070–82.e1.
20. Melvin JS, Stryker LS, Sierra RJ. Tranexamic acid in hip and knee arthroplasty. J Am Acad Orthop Surg 2015;23(12):732–40.
21. Ye W, Liu Y, Liu WF, et al. The optimal regimen of oral tranexamic acid administration for primary total knee/hip replacement: a meta-analysis and narrative review of a randomized controlled trial. J Orthop Surg Res 2020;15(1):457.
22. Wang F, Zhao K-C, Zhao M-M, et al. The efficacy of oral versus intravenous tranexamic acid in reducing blood loss after primary total knee and hip arthroplasty: A meta-analysis. Medicine (Baltimore) 2018;97(36):e12270.
23. Kayupov E, Fillingham YA, Okroj K, et al. Oral and intravenous tranexamic acid are equivalent at reducing blood loss following total hip arthroplasty: a randomized controlled trial. J Bone Joint Surg Am 2017;99(5):373–8.
24. Fillingham YA, Kayupov E, Plummer DR, et al. The James A. Rand Young Investigator's Award: A randomized controlled trial of oral and intravenous tranexamic acid in total knee arthroplasty: the same efficacy at lower cost? J Arthroplasty 2016;31(9):26–30.

25. Pilbrant A, Schannong M, Vessman J. Pharmacokinetics and bioavailability of tranexamic acid. Eur J Clin Pharmacol 1981;20(1):65–72.

26. Ahmed I, Chan JKK, Jenkins P, et al. Estimating the transfusion risk following total knee arthroplasty. Orthopedics 2012;35(10):e1465–71.

27. Basora M, Tió M, Martin N, et al. Should all patients be optimized to the same preoperative hemoglobin level to avoid transfusion in primary knee arthroplasty? Vox Sang 2014;107(2): 148–52.

28. Yeh JZY, Chen JY, Bin Abd Razak HR, et al. Preoperative haemoglobin cut-off values for the prediction of post-operative transfusion in total knee arthroplasty. Knee Surg Sports Traumatol Arthrosc 2016;24(10):3293–8.

29. Thompson GE, Miller RD, Stevens WC, et al. Hypotensive anesthesia for total hip arthroplasty: a study of blood loss and organ function (brain, heart, liver, and kidney). Anesthesiology 1978;48(2):91–6.

30. Sharrock NE, Salvati EA. Hypotensive epidural anesthesia for total hip arthroplasty: a review. Acta Orthop Scand 1996;67(1):91–107.

31. Freeman AK, Thorne CJ, Gaston CL, et al. Hypotensive epidural anesthesia reduces blood loss in pelvic and sacral bone tumor resections. Clin Orthop Relat Res 2017;475(3):634–40.

32. Darwish A, Lui F. Physiology, Colloid Osmotic Pressure. In: Editorial board. Treasure Island, FL: StatPearls. StatPearls Publishing; 2020. p. 1–9. Available at: http://www.ncbi.nlm.nih.gov/books/NBK541067/. Accessed March 31, 2020.

Anterior Supine Intermuscular Total Hip Arthroplasty at an Ambulatory Surgery Center Versus Hospitalization

Cost and Adverse Events

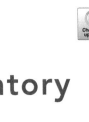

Andrew J. Wodowski, MD[a],
Thomas W. Throckmorton, MD[b],
William M. Mihalko, MD, PhD[b], Patrick C. Toy, MD[b],*

KEYWORDS

- Total hip arthroplasty • Anterior supine intermuscular approach • Ambulatory surgery center
- Costs • Complications

KEY POINTS

- No statistically significant differences were noted in surgery time, blood loss, or complications in anterior supine intermuscular total hip arthroplasty performed at an ambulatory surgery center compared with a hospital setting.
- Length of hospital stay differed significantly between the 2 settings.
- Visual analog scale (VAS) for pain was not significantly different between the 2 settings in the initial postoperative visit; however, a significant difference was noted by the third postoperative visit, with the ambulatory surgery center having a lower VAS for pain than the hospital setting.
- Cost savings were significantly different, with the ambulatory surgery center saving $12,437 over the hospital setting.
- Anterior supine intermuscular total hip arthroplasty at an ambulatory surgery center appears to be as safe as and more cost-effective than performing the procedure in a hospital setting.

Total hip arthroplasty (THA) is an effective and reliable procedure to relieve pain in the hip joint caused by degenerative joint disease and has become one of the most common operations done in the United States.[1,2] Traditionally, hip arthroplasty has been done through a posterior, direct lateral, or anterolateral surgical approach, with inpatient hospital admission. Although these techniques have resulted in good clinical and functional results, even with minimally invasive techniques, multiple muscles may be divided or released off of the proximal femur.[3] As a result, hospital stays may be prolonged because of pain control issues, difficulty with mobilization, individual medical comorbidities, and uncertainty about recovering at home.

Recently, anterior supine intermuscular (ASI) THA has gained popularity in the United States. Proponents of this approach cite a less extensive exposure that uses a true internervous plane

---

[a] OrthoSouth, 2100 Exeter Rd, Germantown, TN 38138, USA; [b] Department of Orthopaedic Surgery & Biomedical Engineering, University of Tennessee-Campbell Clinic, Memphis, TN, USA
* Corresponding author. 1211 Union Avenue, Suite 510, Memphis, TN 38104.
E-mail address: ptoy@campbellclinic.com

Orthop Clin N Am 52 (2021) 209–214
https://doi.org/10.1016/j.ocl.2021.03.011

between the superior gluteal nerve and the femoral nerve, without the need to split or release any muscles.[4] Reports in the literature on ASI THA have shown that this may result in shorter postoperative hospital stays, equivalent functional results, decreased pain, and improved rehabilitation.[5] There also may be substantial cost savings when THA is done as an outpatient rather inpatient procedure.[6]

Surgeons at the authors' institution have been performing ASI THA since 2009 as an inpatient hospital admission and now at the authors' ambulatory surgery center (ASC) since January of 2013. There is an evolving body of literature regarding this surgery center model of hip arthroplasty.[7–13] The purpose of this study was to analyze 1 center's experience with ASI THA by comparing pain scores, complications, and costs of this procedure performed in an ASC to those with the procedure performed in the hospital setting (HS). The authors' hypothesis was that ASC procedures would be more cost-effective than in-hospital THA, with similar rates of complications.

METHODS

After informed consent from all subjects and institutional review board approval, retrospective chart review identified patients who had ASI THA done by the primary author (PCT) between April 2012 and October 2014, for end-stage osteoarthritis of the hip at 1 of 4 locations: 2 ASCs and 2 hospitals. Patients who met the inclusion criteria were contacted by telephone, and the risks and benefits of their voluntary participation in the study were explained. A release of information form was mailed for review and signature. Patients were not included in the financial arm of the study if they did not return their signed release of information form or respond to telephone calls.

Review of records identified 35 patients who had surgery in 1 of the surgery centers and 92 who had their surgery in 1 of the 2 hospitals. These patients varied in medical comorbidities, American Society of Anesthesiologists (ASA) scores, age, status of tobacco use, and body mass index (BMI). To mitigate confounding factors, patients in each group were matched as closely as possible based on these variables. Medical comorbidities and number of medications were identified from medical clearance letters from each patient's primary care physician, if available, and through patient self-reporting of conditions and social history from preoperative office visit health history forms that were available for all patients.

These comorbidities then were evaluated with the Healthcare Cost and Utilization Project Nationwide Inpatient Sample modified Elixhauser Comorbidity Index.[14] This index is a listing of 29 medical comorbidities that have been identified as predictors of outcomes for various health care scenarios. In addition to more common physiologic medical problems, such as diabetes and hypertension, it includes various mental health disorders and substance abuse. This matching process was completed before any further chart review took place and resulted in 35 patients in each group as each ASC patient was matched to a hospital patient for a total of 70 patients in the study. The postoperative protocols for pain control and rehabilitation were identical for patients in both surgical settings. These protocols included multimodal anesthesia without intravenous narcotics and same-day physical therapy (PT) with outpatient PT after discharge.

After the 2 groups were matched, data were obtained from more detailed chart review. Surgical time was defined as documented skin incision time to application of the skin dressing at the close of the case as obtained from operating room records. Postoperative length of stay was measured in hours and was calculated as the time from surgical case stop time to actual discharge time. Total costs of surgery, supplies, and inpatient stay, if applicable, were obtained from patients' explanation of benefits forms obtained from each operative location's billing office. Pain scores were measured by visual analog scale (VAS) or were extrapolated from postoperative office visit notes and PT notes. Mild pain was represented by a VAS equivalent of 1 to 3; moderate pain, 4 to 7; and severe pain, 8 to 10.[15] A complication was defined as any event that caused deviation from a standard postoperative course, such as readmission to the hospital in the first 90 days after surgery, prosthetic joint infection, or need for blood transfusion. Readmission was defined as admission to a hospital or an emergency department visit related to a patient's operation within 90 days after surgery.

All variables were compared and standard statistical calculations for significance were calculated with a computer program (StatPlus:-mac v5, AnalystSoft). Means were compared by analysis of variance functions, and 0.05 was set as the significance level (p) for all calculations.

RESULTS

Demographics and variables were recorded for all patients (Table 1). The results of the patient matching process equalized the groups so there

Table 1
Perioperative characteristics of patient cohorts

	Ambulatory Surgery Center Cohort	Hospital Setting Cohort	P value
Patient factors			
ASA score	2.4	2.5	.86
BMI	29.9 kg/m^2	28.1 kg/m^2	.26
Age	54.3 y	61.4 y	.001
Preoperative HCT	43.8%	41.0%	.002
Surgical factors			
Surgical time	89.2 min	97.7 min	.14
Blood loss	454.3 mL	374.2 mL	.14
Postoperative HCT	34%	31%	.0004
HCT difference	9%	12%	.47
Postoperative LOS	13.4 h	38.0 h	<.01
Outpatient[a]	18 (5.7 h)	6 (6.1 h)	.62
Outcomes			
VAS, first follow-up	2.2	2.7	.13
VAS, third follow-up	0.4	0.8	.03
PT visits	9.8	10.0	.87
Complications	2	4	

Abbreviations: HCT, hematocrit level; HCT difference, difference between preoperative and postoperative hematocrit levels; LOS, length of stay.
[a] Outpatient, defined as discharge on same calendar day as surgery.

were no differences in the number of medical comorbidities or patients who used tobacco. ASA scores and BMI values between the groups did not differ significantly (P = .87 and P = .26, respectively). Patient age was the only variable that was not matched equally between the 2 groups; the patients in the HS group were significantly older, by an average of 7 years (P<.01).

There were no significant differences between the 2 groups in terms of operative time or intraoperative blood loss, but the difference in postoperative hematocrit levels was significant (P = .003) (see Table 1). The average differences between preoperative and postoperative hematocrit levels for the ASC and HS groups were 9.2% and 12.1%, respectively; there was no significant difference between these groups (P = .47). Postoperative hematocrit levels were not available for 11 patients in the ASC group and 7 in the HS group during and after May of 2014, because they purposely were not drawn.

The average postoperative stay was 13.4 hours in the ASC group and 38.0 hours in the HS group; this difference (average of 24.5 h) was significant (P<.01). Eighteen of the

ASC patients (51%) and 6 of the HS patients (17%) were discharged from the surgical facility on the same calendar day as their operation (ie, outpatient surgery). A trend toward a shorter postoperative stay was noted for the outpatients in the ASC group, although the difference was not significant (see Table 1).

At patients' first follow-up office visit (10–14 days after surgery), VAS data were obtained for all ASC patients and all but 2 of the HS patients. At the third postoperative office visit (65–90 d after surgery), VAS data were obtained for 33 of the ASC patients and 34 of the HS patients. There was no significant difference in VAS scores between groups at the first postoperative visit, but a significant difference (P = .03) was noted at the third follow-up appointment (see Table 1). The number of visits to outpatient PT was available for 28 ASC patients and 29 HS patients, and there was no significant difference noted between groups in the number of sessions attended (see Table 1).

Overall, there were few complications (7%). In the ASC group, 1 infection ultimately required revision and 1 blood transfusion of 2 U of packed red blood cells was necessary, both requiring admission to a hospital. The patient requiring transfusion was admitted directly to the hospital from the surgery center in the morning after surgery. In the HS group, 3 blood transfusions, of 2 U each, were required in 3 different patients. One additional patient required readmission to the hospital for gastrointestinal infection a few days after surgery.

For the cost analysis, financial data were available for all 35 ASC patients and 27 of the HS patients (Table 2). The average total cost for ASI THA at an ASC was $29,421.54. The average total cost for the same procedure performed at an inpatient facility was $41,858.60. This represented a cost savings of $12,437 for the ASC group (P<.01). For ASC outpatients, the average cost savings was $7482 compared with the HS outpatients, a significant difference (P<.01) (see Table 2).

DISCUSSION

The ASI THA technique has become popular recently because of its numerous advantages. As a minimally invasive technique,[16] it is an attractive option for many patients. ASI THA uses a true neuromuscular interval and has been shown to cause less muscle damage to the hip abductors than the posterior approach.[17] Component orientation in abduction and anteversion and stem alignment are acceptable and reproducible.[18] One study demonstrated that the ASI approach resulted in a higher percentage of patients discharged home rather than to a rehabilitation center, less narcotic pain medication use, and less use of assistive ambulatory devices compared with traditional posterior THA.[19] Furthermore, the ASI approach has been shown to result in a significant improvement in internal and external range of motion compared with the posterior approach, and functional hip scores are equivalent to or higher than those obtained in similar manner after the posterior or lateral approach for THA.[20–22] Importantly, ASI THA has been suggested to result in a shorter length of stay and fewer dislocations.[5,23–26] Complications of this approach are rare, as they are after THA through a posterior approach, but some studies have shown a slightly higher frequency of fractures and nerve injuries.[16]

The authors found no significant differences in operative time or blood loss, but the postoperative hematocrit level was significantly lower in the HS group even though there was more intraoperative blood loss in the ASC group. Beginning in May of 2014, however, routine postoperative hematocrit evaluation was discontinued. Since that time, none of 11 ASC patients and 6 of 13 HS patients had a postoperative hematocrit drawn. No transfusions have been required since this modification to the postoperative protocol was implemented.

Besides the 1 infection in the ASC group, no complications or readmissions occurred in the last 15 cases for either group. These findings are similar to those of other studies that found an inverse relationship between the number of ASI THA procedures performed and the number of complications,[27–29] suggesting that the safety of the procedure is more dependent on surgeon experience than on surgical setting.

Although there was no significant difference in VAS scores between groups at the first postoperative visit, scores were significantly better in the ASC group at the third follow-up visit. This is similar to outcomes reported by Barrett and colleagues,[28] who described less initial postoperative pain and rapid improvement in VAS pain scores with the ASI approach. Additionally, there was no difference in the number of visits to outpatient PT between groups. One ASC patient refused to attend formal outpatient PT because of how well he performed with PT on the day of his surgery. The reasons for similar numbers of PT visits likely are multifactorial and may include patients' subjective opinions regarding their functional status based on their preoperative expectations and early postoperative course. Because preoperative, intraoperative, and postoperative protocols did not vary between the 2 study groups, performing the operation at an ASC and discharging ambulatory patients on the same day with appropriate medical equipment and pain control appear to be safe. Preoperative education regarding postoperative function, pain expectations, and PT goals is vital to the success of ASC THA.

| Table 2 | | |
| Cost analysis for the 2 patient cohorts | | |
Group	Mean	P value
All ASC	$29,421.54	<.01
All HS	$41,858	
ASC outpatients[a]	$29,724.65	<.01
HS outpatients[a]	$37, 206.75	

[a] Discharged on same calendar day as surgery.

The expenditures of health care dollars per capita in the United States is one of the highest in the world and is an unsettling trend that may be unsustainable for future generations.[30] Current health care economics has shifted focus toward thoughtful use of resources and elimination of frivolous expenditures. The authors' model of ASI THA in an ASC setting resulted in an average cost difference of $12,437, a substantial savings to patients and insurance companies. These results are in agreement with a recent study from the Hospital for Special Surgery, where a difference of approximately $7000 was noted between THA performed in a hospital and in an outpatient surgery center.[6] Comparison of costs between outpatients in the 2 groups found a significant savings of $7,482, suggesting that the ASC model may eliminate some needless expenses, making it more cost-efficient than the HS.

Limitations of the study include the short follow-up, which encompassed the 90-day global period for VAS results and complications. Dislocation, periprosthetic fracture, or thromboembolic episodes may occur later in the postoperative course but studies have shown late complications to be generally similar after ASI THA and standard THA, so no significant differences would be expected at longer-term follow-up.[16,29] This study focused on the immediate results as they pertain to pain as well as complications and cost during this global period. The number of patients in each group is smaller than in other reports but matched with regard to demographics and comorbidities; the authors were not able to match age. Sample size estimation and a power analysis were not performed before the study was begun because the authors included all ASC patients who had surgery during the study time frame. Additionally, not all patients were true outpatients, but this was due to the transition period away from the hospital procedures and into the surgery center. This period evolved out of necessity as the nursing staff, therapists, and operating room staff had to shift away from treating postoperative patients undergoing simple procedures to the relatively more complex procedure of a hip replacement.

Overall, in this matched series, ASI THA at an ASC appears to be as safe as and more cost-effective than performing the procedure in the HS. Longer follow-up of these patients is necessary to confirm that the ASC procedure attains equivalent, if not superior, functional outcomes with fewer complications than standard THA.

CLINICS CARE POINTS

- ASI THA uses a neuromuscular interval that causes less muscle damage to hip abductors than a posterior approach.
- Component orientation and stem alignment are reproducible.
- Reported benefits over a posterior approach include greater range of motion, fewer dislocations, higher functional hip scores, less narcotic pain use, less assistive ambulatory devices needed, and earlier discharge to home.
- Complications of this approach are rare, but a slightly higher frequency of fractures and nerve injuries has been reported.
- Performing ASI THA in an ASC and discharging patients on the same day with appropriate medical equipment and pain control appears safe. The safety of the procedure is more dependent on surgeon experience than surgical setting.
- Preoperative education on postoperative function, pain expectations, and PT goals is necessary.
- ASI THA in an ASC may result in substantial savings.
- Longer follow-up is necessary to confirm equivalent functional outcomes of ASI THA compared with standard THA performed in the HS.

DISCLOSURE

The authors report no conflicts of interest in regard to this work.

REFERENCES

1. Bachmeier CJM, March LM, Cross MJ, et al. A comparison of outcomes in osteoarthritis patients undergoing total hip and knee replacement surgery. Osteoarth Cartilage 2001;9:137–46.
2. Katz JN, Wright EA, Wright J, et al. Twelve-year risk of revision after primary total hip replacement in the U.S. medicare population. J Bone Joint Surg Am 2012;94:1825–32.
3. Pitto RP. CORR Insights: Is limited incision better than standard total hip arthroplasty? A meta-analysis. Clin Orthop Relat Res 2013;471:1295–6.
4. Schweppe ML, Sevler TM, Plate JF, et al. Does surgical approach in total hip arthroplasty affect rehabilitation, discharge disposition, and readmission rate? Surg Technol Int 2013;23:219–27.

5. Dorr LD, Maheshwari AV, Long WT, et al. Early pain relief and function after posterior minimally invasive and conventional total hip arthroplasty. A prospective, randomized, blinded study. J Bone Joint Surg Am 2007;89:1153–60.

6. Avnardi M, Post Z, Ong A, et al. Outpatient surgery as a means of cost reduction in total hip arthroplasty: a case-control study. HSS J 2014;10:252–5.

7. Goyal N, Chen AF, Pedgett SE, et al. Otto Aufranc Award: A multicenter, randomized study of outpatient versus inpatient total hip arthroplasty. Clin Orthop Relat Res 2017;475:364–72.

8. Klein GR, Posner JM, Levine HB, et al. Same day total hip arthroplasty performed at an ambulatory surgical center: 90-day complication rate on 549 patients. J Arthroplasty 2017;32:1103–6.

9. Lovecchio F, Alvi H, Sahota S, et al. Is outpatient arthroplasty as safe as fast-track inpatient arthroplasty? A propensity score matched analysis. J Arthroplasty 2016;31(9 Suppl):197–201.

10. Nelson SJ, Webb ML, Lukasiewica AM, et al. Is outpatient total hip arthroplasty safe? J Arthroplasty 2017;32:1439–42.

11. Parcells BW, Giacobbe D, Macknet D, et al. Total joint arthroplasty in a stand-alone ambulatory surgical center: short-term outcomes. Orthopedics 2016;39:223–8.

12. Springer BD, Odum SM, Vegari DN, et al. Impact of inpatient versus outpatient total joint arthroplasty on 30-day hospital readmission rates and unplanned episodes of care. Orthop Clin North Am 2017;48:15–23.

13. Toy PC, Fournier MN, Throckmorton TW, et al. Low rates of adverse events following ambulatory outpatient total hip arthroplasty at a free-standing surgery center. J Arthroplasty 2017;33:46–50.

14. Browne JA, Novicoff WM, D'Apuzzo MR. Medicaid payer status is associated with in-hospital morbidity and resource utilization following primary total joint arthroplasty. J Bone Joint Surg Am 2014;96:e180.

15. Boonstra AM, Schiphorst Preuper HR, Balk GA, et al. Cut-off points for mild, moderate, and severe pain on the visual analogue scale for pain in patients with chronic musculoskeletal pain. Pain 2014;155:2545–50.

16. Post ZD, Orozco F, Diaz-Ledezma C, et al. Direct anterior approach for total hip arthroplasty: Indications, technique, and results. J Am Acad Orthop Surg 2014;22:595–603.

17. Meneghini RM, Pagnano MW, Trousdale RT, et al. Muscle damage during MIS total hip arthroplasty: Smith-Petersen versus posterior approach. Clin Biomech 2009;24:812–8.

18. Alexandrov T, Ahlmann ER, Menendez LR. Early clinical and radiographic results of minimally invasive anterior approach hip arthroplasty. Adv Orthop 2014;2014:954208.

19. Zawadsky MW, Paulus MC, Murray PJ, et al. Early outcome comparison between the direct anterior approach and the mini-incision posterior approach for primary total hip arthroplasty: 150 consecutive cases. J Arthroplasty 2014;29:1256–60.

20. Paraskevopoulos A, Marenghi P, Alesci M, et al. Mini-invasive anterior approach in total hip arthroplasty: short-term follow-up. Acta Biomed 2014;85:75–80.

21. Taunton MJ, Mason JB, Odum SM, et al. Direct anterior total hip arthroplasty yields more rapid voluntary cessation of all walking aids: a prospective, randomized clinical trial. J Arthroplasty 2014;29(9 Suppl):169–72.

22. Mirza AJ, Lombardi AV Jr, Morris MJ, et al. A mini-anterior approach to the hip for total joint replacement: optimizing results: improving hip joint replacement outcomes. Bone Joint J 2014;96-B(11 Suppl A):32–5.

23. Higgins BT, Barlow DR, Heagerty NE, et al. Anterior vs. posterior approach for total hip arthroplasty, a systematic review and meta-analysis. J Arthroplasty 2015;30:419–34.

24. Siguier T, Siguier M, Brumpt B. Mini-incision anterior approach does not increase dislocation rate: a study of 1037 total hip replacements. Clin Orthop Relat Res 2004;426:164–73.

25. Martin CT, Pugely AJ, Gao Y, et al. A comparison of hospital length of stay and short-term morbidity between the anterior and the posterior approaches to total hip arthroplasty. J Arthroplasty 2013;28:849–54.

26. Müller DA, Zingg PO, Dora C. Anterior minimally invasive approach for total hip replacement: five-year survivorship and learning curve. Hip Int 2014;24:277–83.

27. De Geest T, Vansintian P, De Loore G. Direct anterior total hip arthroplasty: complications and early outcome in a series of 300 cases. Acta Orthop Belg 2013;79:166–73.

28. Barrett WP, Turner SE, Leopold JP. Prospective randomized study of direct anterior vs posterolateral approach for total hip arthroplasty. J Arthroplasty 2013;28:1634–8.

29. Berend KR. The mini-anterior approach: optimises THA outcome – affirms. Bone Joint J 2014;96-B(suppl):8–21.

30. Sawyer B, Cox C. How does health spending in the U.S. compare to other countries?. Available at: https://www.healthsystemtracker.org/chart-collection/health-spending-u-s-compare-countries/#item-start. Accessed June 28, 2018.

Trauma

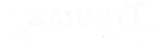

Malrotation of Long Bones

Matthew Sullivan, MD[a], Kelsey Bonilla, MD[b],
Derek Donegan, MD, MBA[c],*

KEYWORDS
• Intramedullary nail • Malrotation • Femoral fractures • Tibial fractures • Osteotomy • Intramedullary fixation • Postoperative complication

KEY POINTS
• Malrotation occurs in 15% to 40% of femoral fractures and 20% to 40% of tibial fractures treated with intramedullary fixation.
• Computed tomography is the gold standard for calculating rotation in cases of suspected rotational malreduction; clinical examination is not a reliable method for assessing rotation.
• Malrotation can often be prevented with careful attention to intraoperative radiographs and awareness of risk factors.
• Intraoperative femoral and tibial rotation can be confirmed by matching contralateral version or use of the cortical step sign.
• Cases of malrotation can be corrected with derotation before fracture union or with intramedullary or open osteotomy following symptomatic malunion.

INTRODUCTION

Incidence

Malunion is a well-known complication of intramedullary nailing of long bone fractures. Although much attention is paid to coronal and sagittal plane deformities, malrotation tends to be underreported despite being associated with significant morbidity. Postoperative malrotation of the femur, typically defined as a difference in anteversion of 15° or more compared with contralateral side,[1–3] is evident in up to 27.6% of femoral shaft fractures and up to 40% of subtrochanteric femur fractures treated with intramedullary stabilization.[1,4,5] When malrotation is defined as greater than a 10° difference from the contralateral femur, the incidence has been reported to be as high as 40% to 50%.[6–8] Despite the fact that tibial rotation is often considered easier to assess, the incidence of rotational malreduction of tibial shaft fractures beyond 10° following treatment with intramedullary devices has been reported to be between 22% and 41%.[9–12]

Functional Implications

Much of the reason for the underreporting of postoperative torsional deformities is likely related to the patient's ability to tolerate a significant amount of malrotation through compensatory action of adjacent joints, which results in a large proportion of asymptomatic cases.[7,13–16] It has long been reported that malrotation affects the development of osteoarthritis; however, findings related to functional outcome measures are often unclear or inconsistent due to variability in choice of outcome scores and manner in which rotation is measured.[17]

Despite this, femoral malrotation has been associated with difficulty with specific activities such as running, stairs, and sports, which has been suggested to be related to increased patellofemoral contact stresses.[6,8,15,18,19] Others have used computer-generated models to demonstrate that malrotation at various levels of the femur produces malalignment of the mechanical axis in the sagittal and coronal planes,

[a] SUNY Upstate, 6620 Fly Road, Suite 200, East Syracuse, NY 13057, USA; [b] Department of Orthopaedics, University of Pennsylvania, 3737 Market Street, 6th Floor, Philadelphia, PA 19104, USA; [c] Department of Orthoapedics, Division of Orthopaedic Trauma, University of Pennsylvania, 3737 Market Street, 6th Floor, Philadelphia, PA 19104, USA
* Corresponding author.
E-mail address: derek.donegan@pennmedicine.upenn.edu

Orthop Clin N Am 52 (2021) 215–229
https://doi.org/10.1016/j.ocl.2021.03.008

which produces a medial or lateral shift in the center of force through the knee.[20–22] Similarly, malrotation of the tibiotalar joint beyond 10° produces joint incongruity, which decreases the area over which load is transmitted across the articular surface, and internal or external malrotation beyond 20° increases peak pressures across the articular surface.[23]

It seems that patients tolerate internal rotation deformities of the femur better than external rotation due to their ability to compensate with gait.[8,15] However, others have not detected differences in functional outcomes scores or knee pain in patients with postoperative femoral or tibial malrotation, which suggests that some patients are able to adequately compensate for the deformity.[2,11,14,24]

Risk Factors

Fracture location is a risk factor for coronal and sagittal plane deformities; however, it has not been routinely proved to be a risk factor for torsional deformity.[6,8,25] A notable exception to this is subtrochanteric femur fractures, which are at risk of internal rotation malrotation due to the deforming forces on the proximal and distal fracture fragments.[1,3,5] Transverse, segmental, and comminuted fracture patterns and those associated with bone loss are also considered to be at high risk of malrotation, although several studies have challenged the notion that fracture comminution is a predictor of malrotation.[1,7,26,27] Similarly patient factors such as age, sex, and body mass index and surgeon factors including fellowship training, choice of antegrade or retrograde nail, decision to fix associated fibula fractures, and daytime versus nighttime surgery have not been shown to have a significant impact on postoperative malrotation.[7,12,26–29]

Interestingly, freehand drilling of distal interlock screws induces an average of 5.8° of malrotation due to contact between the drill passing through the locking hole in the nail off axis, which suggests that computer-navigated placement of interlocks can help prevent inadvertent deformity.[30] There is also debate surrounding the effect that use of a fracture table versus manual traction has on postoperative malrotation, with some suggesting fracture tables increase risk of internal rotation deformities[31]; this occurs when the distal segment is internally rotated relative to the femoral head and neck, resulting in an increase in femoral anteversion and an internally rotated foot on the injured side. The risk of internal rotation malreduction that can occur while applying traction and

internal rotation to the limb on a fracture table is further exacerbated by the deforming forces on pertrochanteric hip fractures. Fortunately, this has not been routinely reproduced, suggesting that awareness of this tendency can help prevent malrotation.[26]

Prevention

Much of the challenge with obtaining proper rotational alignment is related to the difficulty associated with obtaining adequate fluoroscopic images intraoperatively. Because there is very little remodeling that occurs in the axial plane, it is critical to establish proper rotation at the time of fixation.[32] Comparison to the uninjured extremity by clinical examination is not a reliable method of preventing rotational malalignment, leading to malrotation greater than 20° in 42% to 62% of patients examined supine.[1,8,33] Computed tomography (CT) is the gold standard for measuring rotation of both the femur and tibia in the axial plane.[34,35] Although preoperative cross-sectional imaging is not routinely necessary, CT scans are often performed on polytrauma patients to assess for other injuries. When this information is available, measurements of the contralateral extremity can be calculated preoperatively to ensure proper rotational alignment of the injured extremity at the time of surgery.

Fluoroscopic technique

Several methods for judging femoral rotation intraoperatively have been described, most of which depend on normal anatomy of the uninjured contralateral limb. Matching the profile of the contralateral lesser trochanter has been shown to be a reliable reference for judging femoral rotation, leading to less than 5° of malrotation with good interobserver reliability.[9,36,37]

Others have described methods of measuring anteversion of the contralateral hip intraoperatively and then matching this when locking rotation of the nail. Tornetta and colleagues determine version of the uninjured hip by calculating the difference between a true lateral of the knee, judged by overlap of the posterior cortices of the distal femoral condyles, and a true lateral of the hip. The distal fracture fragment is then rotated to reproduce this version and locked in place. This technique resulted in malrotation of less than 5° judged by postoperative CT.[16]

Bråten and colleagues also describe a technique that involves obtaining a perfect lateral of the knee and then, without rotating the c-arm, imaging the proximal femur at a 30° to

60° angle to the long axis of the femur. The resulting neck-horizontal angle has been shown to closely estimate femoral anteversion of the uninjured extremity. The proximal and distal fracture fragments can then be rotated to this relative position and statically locked to mimic the version of the contralateral limb.[38]

With respect to tibial fractures, the rotational profile of the uninjured limb can also be determined intraoperatively and then reproduced before statically locking the injured side. One technique to measure the torsion of the uninjured extremity involves obtaining a perfect lateral of the knee and then, without moving the limb, rotating the c-arm at the level of the ankle to obtain a tangential view of the articular surface medial malleolus.[9,39,40] Unfortunately these methods cannot be used in the setting of bilateral injury patterns or contralateral deformity.

Caution must be used when using techniques that rely on the contralateral extremity because femoral anteversion has been shown to differ by 11.8° between limbs.[41] The cortical step sign is another technique to assess rotation, which does not rely on mimicking the anatomy of the contralateral limb. Differences in the cortical widths of the fracture fragments indicate rotational malreduction because cortical thickness varies about the longitudinal axis of the femur, with the imaged thickness of both the medial and lateral cortices decreasing with either internal or external rotation.[42] This technique can also be used to judge rotation of tibial shaft fractures because the medial and lateral cortices of the tibia project different thicknesses with rotation.[9] This technique can be particularly useful for transverse fracture patterns; however, it cannot be used in fractures with extensive bone loss or comminution.

Other techniques

Although standard fluoroscopy is undoubtedly the most commonly used tool for assessing rotation intraoperatively, other methods have been described. A recent study using a sawbones model of transverse femoral shaft fractures demonstrated that 3-dimensional (3D) c-arm produces significantly more accurate measurements of femoral version than standard fluoroscopy.[43] And what is perhaps more of a historical note, ultrasound can be used to estimate femoral anteversion and has been shown to correlate well with CT measurements.[44]

Goals

Ultimately, malrotation is still a relatively common and underreported complication of the

treatment of long bone fractures with an intramedullary nail. Here, 3 such cases are reviewed, and the various techniques used to correct the resulting deformities are described.

CASES

Case 1: Pertrochanteric Malrotation

Presentation

The patient is a 57-year-old otherwise healthy woman who presented to clinic as a new referral complaining of persistent groin pain, feelings of motion at the fracture site, an internally rotated foot, and a leg length discrepancy. Ten months prior she sustained a fall, resulting in a minimally displaced intertrochanteric femur fracture with varus malalignment (**Fig. 1**). She was subsequently taken to the operating room and treated with a short cephalomedullary hip fracture nail. Surgery was performed on a fracture table. Intraoperative fluoroscopy highlights the extent of internal rotation of the femoral shaft, which is evident with the lack of a lesser trochanteric profile on the anteroposterior view (**Fig. 2**). Surgery was tolerated well and the postoperative course was uneventful; however, she states that she never "felt right" after surgery.

Because of lack of satisfaction with her hip function the patient sought a second opinion 10 months following surgery. The patient reported no significant medical comorbidities and noted a well-functioning and painless ipsilateral total knee arthroplasty, which was placed several years prior. Examination of the patient demonstrated a marked Trendelenburg gait. She had pain with log roll and was unable to perform a straight leg raise secondary to pain.

Deformity measurements

Plain film radiographs at that time demonstrated a broken cephalomedullary short hip fracture nail with varus malalignment of the proximal femur (**Fig. 3**A, B). Because of the high index of suspicion for rotational malalignment a CT scanogram of the bilateral lower extremities was obtained, which also demonstrated the intertrochanteric nonunion (**Fig. 3**C). Determination of femoral version/rotation is performed by measuring the angle between the posterior condylar axis of the knee and the long axis of the femoral neck. The version of the injured hip is 33° of anteversion, whereas this patient's native version is −10° anteversion (**Fig. 4**). Total rotational malalignment of injured to uninjured extremities is 43°, which explains the internal rotation deformity of the injured side compared to the contralateral side. The coronal plane deformity was also identified before revision

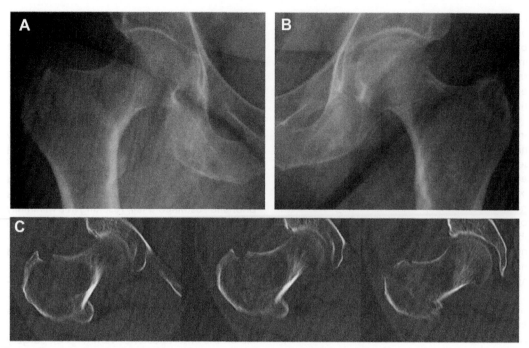

Fig. 1. Fracture pattern at the time of injury. (*A*) Minimally displaced intertrochanteric fracture of right hip compared with (*B*) uninjured left hip. (*C*) CT cuts demonstrating fracture morphology.

and was determined to be 21° of varus angulation (Fig. 5).

A thorough nonunion workup was undertaken, in order to identify any additional treatable causes for this failure. Inflammatory markers were unremarkable, as were endocrine and other metabolic laboratories, which can be implicated in nonunions. As such, this nonunion was determined to be the result of an unfavorable mechanical environment generated by the 43° malrotation deformity.

Operative technique

The patient was offered 2 options for surgical management. The first was hardware removal and total hip arthroplasty. The second was hardware removal, subtrochanteric osteotomy, and blade plate insertion following multiplanar deformity correction. The patient opted for the latter.

Preoperative planning was critical to successful execution of this complex malnonunion repair. Once the deformity was identified, 43° of malrotation and 21° of varus angulation, the

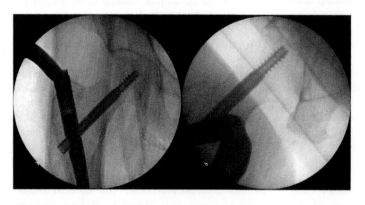

Fig. 2. Intraoperative fluoroscopy at index procedure. Two views of hip demonstrate internal rotation of the femoral shaft with absence of lesser trochanter profile.

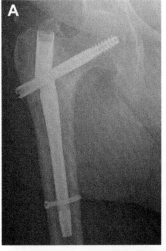
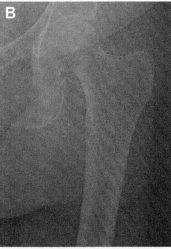
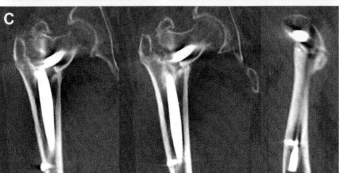

Fig. 3. Imaging obtained 10 months postoperatively. (A) AP image of left proximal femur demonstrating broken cephalomedullary nail and varus malalignment. (B) Contralateral hip demonstrating native coronal plane alignment, and two views of hip demonstrate internal rotation of the femoral shaft with absence of lesser trochanter profile. (C) Coronal CT cuts depicting fracture nonunion. AP, anteroposterior.

authors commenced planning the location of the osteotomy, location of blade plate insertion, and method by which rotation would be corrected. A 95° angled blade plate was chosen in order to obtain maximal compression across the osteotomy. Fig. 6 demonstrates the location and orientation of the subtrochanteric osteotomy as well as the insertion point and final resting position of the blade.

The rotation was corrected using a 4-mm Schanz pin in the proximal femur, and a parallel pin was placed in the distal femur. These were placed before the osteotomy was performed. Once the blade plate was applied, these wires

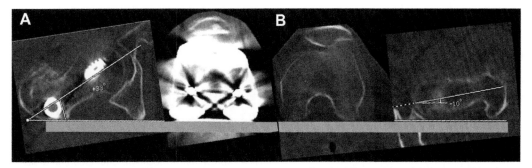

Fig. 4. Calculation of proximal femoral malrotation. (A) Version of injured hip measured to be 33° of anteversion using Hernandez method by calculating the angle between a line connecting the center of the femoral head and neck and the posterior distal femoral condylar axis. (B) Native alignment of contralateral hip measured to be 10° of retroversion, resulting in a 43° rotational discrepancy.

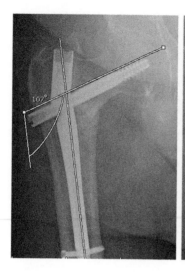
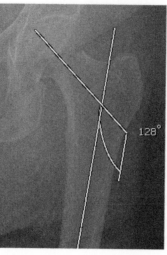

Fig. 5. Calculation of coronal malalignment. Injured extremity noted to be in 21° of varus compared with the contralateral hip.

were used to measure 43° of rotational correction with the aid of an assistant at the end of the operating room table using a goniometer (Fig. 7).

The extremity was clinically evaluated for rotational correction before arousal from anesthesia and demonstrated clear improvement in symmetry compared with preoperative alignment (Fig. 8). The fracture went onto union following correction of the mechanical environment, and the patient's pain resolved and her gait returned to normal by 6 months postoperatively (Fig. 9).

Case 2: Femoral Shaft Malrotation
Presentation
The patient is a 15-year-old boy who was a pedestrian struck by an automobile. He presented to a community hospital with a closed comminuted proximal diaphyseal femur fracture (Fig. 10). The patient was otherwise healthy and had no other traumatic injuries. He was urgently taken to the operating room for open reduction and medullary fixation of his injury. A piriformis entry antegrade femoral nail was used and an open anatomic reduction was attempted. Postoperative flat plate images point to several technical issues that occurred intraoperatively (Fig. 11). The overall alignment of the femur is that of varus and apex anterior angulation. This characteristic deformity is a result of a start point that is too lateral and anterior. The surgeon then attempted to correct the varus alignment by performing an open approach and placing a cerclage cable; however, this did not produce the desired outcome. The patient was subsequently transferred to the trauma center for further management.

Deformity measurements
On arrival, CT scans of bilateral lower extremities were obtained in order to assess rotational alignment, as a malreduction was suspected. Measurements of the bilateral femoral necks and posterior distal femoral condyles demonstrate an 18° anteversion deformity of the affected side due to internal rotation of the distal fragment (Fig. 12). A discussion was

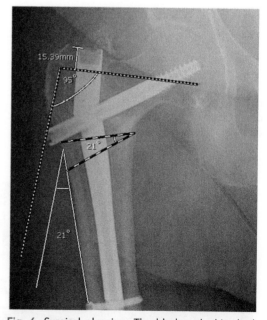

Fig. 6. Surgical planning. The black and white hash line represents the location, orientation, and size of the osteotomy needed to correct varus deformity. The dotted black and white line represents the blade plate orientation, insertion point, and final resting position in the femoral head.

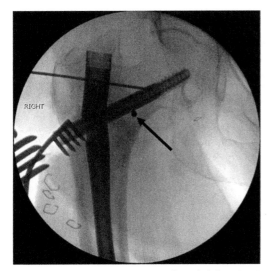

Fig. 7. Intraoperative correction of axial deformity. A 4.0-mm Schanz pin is placed in the proximal femur (*arrow*), and a corresponding pin was placed in the distal femur (not shown). These pins were placed perfectly parallel to one another and used to assess rotational correction with the assistance of a goniometer.

undertaken with the patient and family, and the decision was made to perform a rotational correction only. Given his age, the authors felt strongly that his varus malreduction would not hinder union or function. As such, the patient was taken to the operating room for rotational correction.

Surgical technique
With the CT scan to guide the degree of correction that needed to be obtained, 4-mm Schanz pins were placed proximal and distal to the fracture in perfect parallel orientation (Fig. 13). The distal interlocking bolts were then removed. The limb was then derotated by approximately 20°,

and new interlocking bolts were placed. Rotational correction is confirmed by an unscrubbed assistant who stands at the end of the table with a goniometer and clinical correction of rotation is confirmed after the drapes are removed (Fig. 14). The patient presented for final follow-up 10 months after surgery with complete union and clinical rotational symmetry (Fig. 15).

Both of these cases involving femoral malrotation were performed on a fracture table, which increases the risk of internal rotation malreduction if careful attention is not paid to other markers of version. It is important to be aware of this tendency and be familiar with multiple techniques to confirm rotation in order to avoid this complication.

Case 3: Tibial Shaft Malrotation
Presentation
The patient is a 38-year-old male smoker who sustained a tibial shaft fracture that went on to nonunion following treatment with an intramedullary nail. The fracture successfully healed after revision open reduction and internal fixation with autograft. He underwent removal of hardware but continued to have knee pain and difficulty with running, stairs, and ambulation. He presented to us 2.5 years after his original injury for a second opinion, with radiographs demonstrating a healed fracture with malrotation deformity (Fig. 16). CT scan at that time was obtained, and a 31° external rotation deformity was measured by radiology.

Deformity measurement
Tibial torsion can be calculated as the angle between the proximal and distal tibial axes (Fig. 17). The proximal tibial axis is defined as the tangent line to the proximal tibial plateau. The bimalleolar axis is the most reliable method for measuring the distal tibial axis and can be

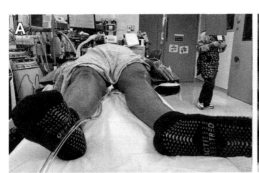
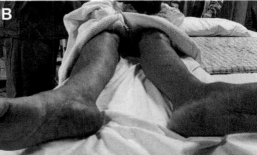

Fig. 8. Preoperative and postoperative clinical photos. (*A*) Asymmetric version evident preoperatively with marked internal rotation of right limb. (*B*) Limb alignment following revision fixation.

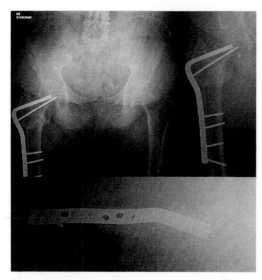

Fig. 9. Postoperative imaging demonstrating fracture union. Radiographs obtained at 6-month follow-up demonstrates osteotomy union and anatomic correction of the proximal femur.

determined by connecting the center of the medial and lateral malleoli just distal to the plafond on a CT cut where the talus is visible.[35] Right tibial torsion was calculated to be 50.4° and left tibial torsion measured 25.9°, resulting in a 24.5° external rotation deformity of the right tibia compared with the uninjured extremity.

Operative technique

Based on these measurements and the patient's symptoms, the decision was made to go to the operating room for derotational osteotomy. A suprapatellar approach to the patellofemoral joint was used, and the appropriate start point was identified under fluoroscopic guidance. After placement of the guidewire, a 0.016 K-wire was placed in the tibial tubercle and, using a sterile goniometer, another was placed in the distal metaphysis 31° externally rotated to the first. A portion of his prior incision was opened over the metaphyseal-diaphyseal junction, and dissection was carried down subperiosteally. The bone was marked with a bovie above and below the level of the planned osteotomy site. A microsagittal saw was used to perform the osteotomy, and the ball tip guide wire was passed beyond the osteotomy into the physeal scar of the distal tibia. The tibia was then reamed sequentially up to 11.5 mm, and a nail of an appropriate length of 10 mm was inserted and

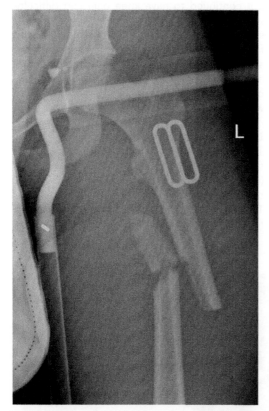

Fig. 10. Injury radiograph. AP of the proximal femoral shaft obtained immediately after the injury demonstrated a closed left comminuted proximal diaphyseal femoral shaft fracture.

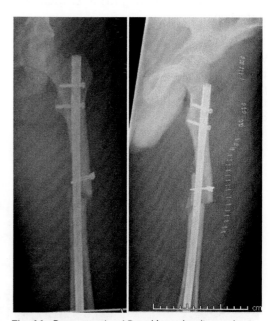

Fig. 11. Postoperative AP and lateral radiographs. Immediate postoperative images demonstrate a varus and apex-anterior flexion malreduction of the femur with an improperly placed piriformis femoral nail.

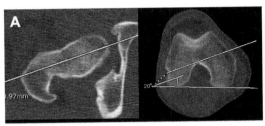
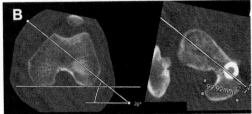

Fig. 12. Calculation of femoral malrotation. (A) CT images of bilateral lower extremities demonstrate native version of 20° of anteversion. (B) Measurements of the left lower extremity confirm an 18° internal rotation malreduction of the fracture. Surgically introduced version of this patient is 38°.

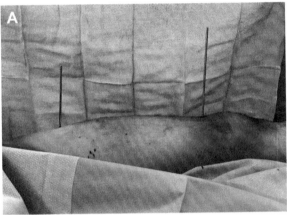
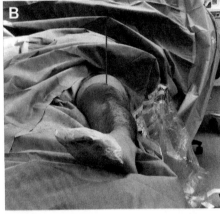

Fig. 13. Intraoperative deformity correction. (A) Before removal of the distal interlocking bolts, 4-mm Schanz pins are placed above and below the fracture. (B) Pins are in perfect parallel orientation to permit accurate correction using a goniometer.

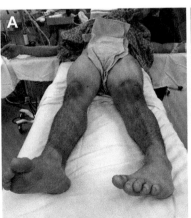
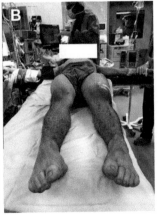

Fig. 14. Preoperative and postoperative clinical images. (A) Preoperatively, a marked internal rotation deformity of the left lower extremity in comparison to the uninjured extremity is present. (B) Derotation results in improved alignment and symmetric appearance of lower extremities.

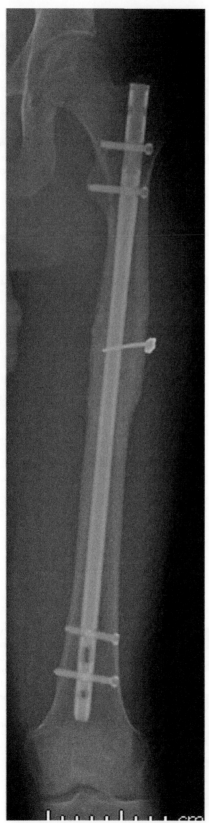

Fig. 15. Postoperative AP of the femur. Imaging 10 months postoperatively demonstrate complete bony union.

locked distally. With the proximal segment unlocked, the distal tibia was internally rotated until the K-wires were parallel (Fig. 18). The bovie marks were evaluated to confirm a 31° change in rotation, and the nail was then compressed and locked proximally through the jig. Rotation was confirmed fluoroscopically before leaving the operating room. The patient was made weight-bearing as tolerated and had significant relief of his symptoms. Radiographs were obtained at regular intervals in the office, and his fracture had successfully united 6 months postoperatively (Fig. 19).

DISCUSSION

Rotational malreduction of long bone fractures is a relatively common complication associated with locked intramedullary nails. Historically, the incidence of malrotation has been underreported. The reasons for this are multifactorial, including inaccurate measurements of rotational profiles on clinical examination, attributing postoperative symptoms to sequela of the original injury as opposed to malrotation, and relatively good ability to compensate for significant rotational deformity.

If malrotation is suspected postoperatively, the rotational profile of the uninjured contralateral limb should be determined before proceeding with any corrective procedure. CT is recognized as the gold standard for measuring femoral and tibial malreduction in the axial plane. Nevertheless, many different axes along which femoral anteversion and tibial torsion can be measured have been described.

The 2 common methods of calculating femoral anteversion on CT are the Hernandez and Weiner methods. The former defines the femoral neck axis as a line connecting the center of the femoral head to the midpoint of the femoral neck on an axial cut of the proximal femur that contains the head, neck, and superior aspect of the greater trochanter. The latter uses a line passing through the middle of the femoral neck where the dorsal and ventral cortices of the neck are parallel to each other. Anteversion is then calculated as this angle relative to the distal femoral condylar axis. Liodakis and colleagues found the Hernandez method to have better intraobserver and interobserver reliability than the Weiner method for determining femoral anteversion in a retrospective analysis of lower extremity rotational profiles.[35]

Tibial torsion can be calculated as the angle between the proximal tibial axis and the distal tibial axis, which can be measured in several

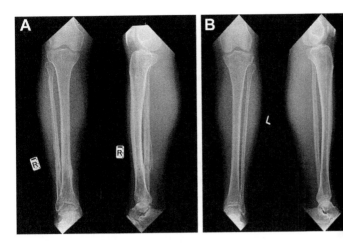

Fig. 16. Preoperative AP and lateral radiographs. (A) Imaging at the time of presentation demonstrates subtle healed malunion of right tibia, as evidenced by asymmetric distal tibiofibular overlap. (B) Imaging of uninjured left tibia for comparison.

different manners (see Fig. 20).[10,45] The Ulm technique defines the distal tibial axis as a line between the center of 2 ellipses, one created by the incisura fibularis and the other by the medial malleolus. The Jend method uses a line connecting the midpoint of a line between the ventral and dorsal corners of the incisura fibularis and the center of a circle formed by the dorsal and ventral corners of the incisura fibularis and the tibial plafond. Finally, the bimalleolar axis, as described previously, connects the center of the medial and lateral malleoli just distal to the tibial plafond. The bimalleolar axis has the greatest intraobserver and interobserver reliability of the 3 methods described.[35]

Once the desired rotational profile has been established, the degree and direction of malrotation of the injured extremity is calculated and

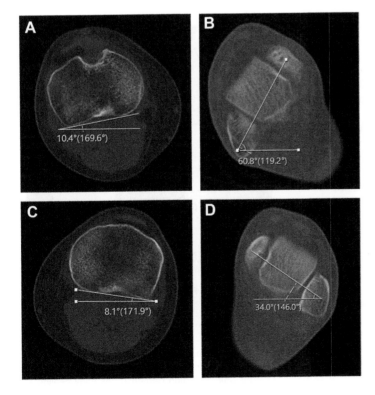

Fig. 17. The author's measurements of preoperative tibial torsional deformity. (A) Right tibial plateau rotation measured at 10.4° and (B) right distal tibial rotation measured at 60.8° determined by the bimalleolar axis, giving right tibial torsion of 50.4°. (C) Left tibial plateau rotation measured at 8.1° and (D) left distal tibial rotation measured at 34.0°, resulting in left tibial torsion of 25.9°. The right tibia was approximately 24.5° externally rotated compared with the uninjured extremity.

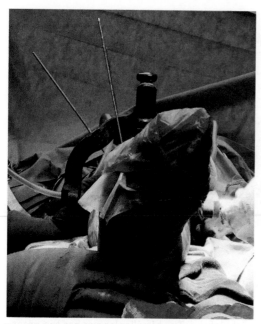

Fig. 18. Intraoperative photo following correction of malrotation. After performing the osteotomy, the distal tibia was internally rotated until the wires in the proximal and distal tibia were superimposed, which reflected a 31° correction (Note: the wire in the 11 o'clock position was used to stabilize handle of the jig to the distal femur and is not relevant to the correction demonstrated).

Some have described performing a circumferential osteotomy with a Gigli saw while maintaining the nail, then removing the interlocks to derotate by the planned amount.[49] A similar minimally invasive technique has been described for the tibia, in which the surgeon uses a drill to perforate the cortex around the retained nail and then completes the cut with an osteotome.[50] Alternatively, open osteotomy can be performed, and a custom 3D-printed jig can be used to ensure accurate correction, after which a new intramedullary nail can be placed.[51]

In most situations the deformity can be corrected all at once; however, it is important to be aware that acute injuries can occur if too great of a correction is attempted in the setting of an old deformity. Corrections that are too aggressive can result in neurologic injury or compartment syndrome, particularly with respect to proximal tibial fractures. When large corrections are undertaken distal to the knee, consideration should be given to peroneal nerve release and prophylactic fasciotomies.

The maximum rotational femoral deformity that should be acutely corrected is 45°, and acute corrections of tibial deformities should not exceed 35° of isolated rotation or 45° of total rotational, sagittal, and coronal

the patient can be taken to the operating room for derotation. Before removing interlocks or performing an osteotomy, it is important to place Steinmann pins on either side of the fracture or planned osteotomy site to serve as markers for correction. Pins can be placed parallel and rotated intraoperatively using a sterile goniometer to measure the correction. Alternatively, pins can be placed at the intended correction angle relative to each other and then rotated until they are aligned.

When malrotation is caught early, the distal interlock can simply be removed allowing for derotation through the fracture site.[34] In the setting of a healed fracture, several techniques for derotation have been described. A minimally invasive technique involves use of an intramedullary saw to produce an osteotomy following removal of the nail; this has the benefit of avoiding soft tissue disruption around the osteotomy site, which ideally protects blood supply to the area while minimizing opportunities for infection.[46–48] It is important to note that replacing an intramedullary form of fixation with an extramedullary method results in disruption of both intramedullary and periosteal blood supply.[49]

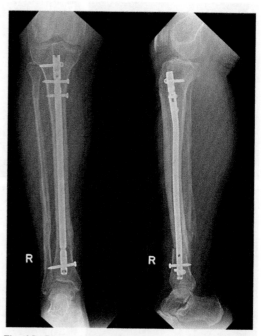

Fig. 19. Postoperative AP and lateral radiographs. Imaging obtained in the office 6 weeks status after repair of right tibia malunion demonstrates early healing in improved position.

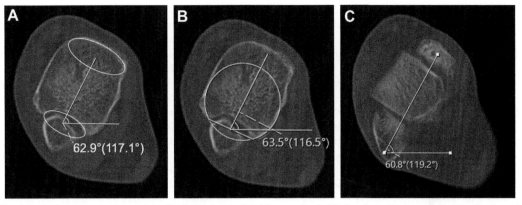

Fig. 20. Techniques to determine distal tibial axis. (*A*) Ulm method, (*B*) Jend method, and (*C*) bimalleolar axis method.

deformity.[48,52] If the required correction is too great to perform all at once, gradual correction can be performed with the application of an external fixator or an Ilizarov fixator.[53,54] Alternatively, acute shortening can be performed in conjunction with deformity correction with planned lengthening at a later time.

SUMMARY

Rotational malreduction is a common postoperative complication following intramedullary nailing of long bone fractures. Here the authors report on 3 cases of malrotation of the femur and the tibia and techniques for postoperative deformity correction. In most situations, this can be prevented at the time of initial surgery with meticulous preoperative planning and careful use of intraoperative fluoroscopy. However, rotational alignment remains difficult to assess by clinical examination, so a high index of suspicion is always necessary, and CT should be obtained if there is concern for rotational malreduction.

CLINICS CARE POINTS

- Malrotation occurs in 15% to 40% of femoral fractures and 20% to 40% of tibial fractures treated with intramedullary fixation.
- CT is the gold standard for calculating rotation in cases of suspected rotational malreduction; clinical examination is not a reliable technique.

- Intraoperative femoral rotation can be confirmed by comparing version to contralateral side, matching the profile of the lesser trochanters, and use of the cortical step sign; intraoperative tibial rotation can be confirmed by matching to the uninjured contralateral side or by use of the cortical step sign.
- Cases of malrotation that are caught early can be corrected with derotation before fracture union or with intramedullary or open osteotomy following symptomatic malunion.
- Malrotation can often be prevented with careful attention to intraoperative radiographs and awareness of risk factors for malreduction, such as use of a fracture table.

DISCLOSURE

M. Sullivan: paid consultant for Depuy Synthes; AOTrauma paid speaker. K. Bonilla: nothing to disclose. D. Donegan: paid consultant for Depuy Synthes, Stryker, and Zimmer Biomet; AOTrauma paid speaker; cofounder and managing partner for ORtelligence Inc.

REFERENCES

1. Lindsey JD, Krieg JC. Femoral malrotation following intramedullary nail fixation. J Am Acad Orthop Surg 2011;19(1):17–26.
2. Kim TY, Lee YB, Chang JD, et al. Torsional malalignment, how much significant in the trochanteric fractures? Injury 2015;46(11):2196–200.
3. Mavrogenis AF, Panagopoulos GN, Megaloikonomos PD, et al. Complications after hip nailing for fractures. Orthopedics 2016;39(1):e108–16.

4. Yang KH, Han DY, Jahng JS, et al. Prevention of malrotation deformity in femoral shaft fracture. J Orthop Trauma 1998;12(8):558–62.

5. Ramanoudjame M, Guillon P, Dauzac C, et al. CT evaluation of torsional malalignment after intertrochanteric fracture fixation. Orthop Traumatol Surg Res 2010;96(8):844–8.

6. Karaman O, Ayhan E, Kesmezacar H, et al. Rotational malalignment after closed intramedullary nailing of femoral shaft fractures and its influence on daily life. Eur J Orthop Surg Traumatol 2014;24(7):1243–7.

7. Bråten M, Terjesen T, Rossvoll I. Torsional deformity after intramedullary nailing of femoral shaft fractures. Measurement of anteversion angles in 110 patients. J Bone Joint Surg Br 1993;75(5):799–803.

8. Jaarsma RL, Pakvis DF, Verdonschot N, et al. Rotational malalignment after intramedullary nailing of femoral fractures. J Orthop Trauma 2004;18(7):403–9.

9. Krettek C, Miclau T, Grün O, et al. Intraoperative control of axes, rotation and length in femoral and tibial fractures. Technical note. Injury 1998;29(Suppl 3):C29–39.

10. Puloski S, Romano C, Buckley R, et al. Rotational malalignment of the tibia following reamed intramedullary nail fixation. J Orthop Trauma 2004;18(7):397–402.

11. Theriault B, Turgeon AF, Pelet S. Functional impact of tibial malrotation following intramedullary nailing of tibial shaft fractures. J Bone Joint Surg Am 2012;94(22):2033–9.

12. Jafarinejad AE, Bakhshi H, Haghnegahdar M, et al. Malrotation following reamed intramedullary nailing of closed tibial fractures. Indian J Orthop 2012;46(3):312–6.

13. Gugala Z, Qaisi YT, Hipp JA, et al. Long-term functional implications of the iatrogenic rotational malalignment of healed diaphyseal femur fractures following intramedullary nailing. Clin Biomech (Bristol, Avon) 2011;26(3):274–7.

14. van der Schoot DK, Den Outer AJ, Bode PJ, et al. Degenerative changes at the knee and ankle related to malunion of tibial fractures. 15-year follow-up of 88 patients. J Bone Joint Surg Br 1996;78(5):722–5.

15. Jaarsma RL, Ongkiehong BF, Grüneberg C, et al. Compensation for rotational malalignment after intramedullary nailing for femoral shaft fractures. An analysis by plantar pressure measurements during gait. Injury 2004;35(12):1270–8.

16. Tornetta P, Ritz G, Kantor A. Femoral torsion after interlocked nailing of unstable femoral fractures. J Trauma 1995;38(2):213–9.

17. Eckhoff DG. Effect of limb malrotation on malalignment and osteoarthritis. Orthop Clin North Am 1994;25(3):405–14.

18. Dagneaux L, Allal R, Pithioux M, et al. Femoral malrotation from diaphyseal fractures results in changes in patellofemoral alignment and higher patellofemoral stress from a finite element model study. Knee 2018;25(5):807–13.

19. Lee TQ, Anzel SH, Bennett KA, et al. The influence of fixed rotational deformities of the femur on the patellofemoral contact pressures in human cadaver knees. Clin Orthop Relat Res 1994;(302):69–74.

20. Gugenheim JJ, Probe RA, Brinker MR. The effects of femoral shaft malrotation on lower extremity anatomy. J Orthop Trauma 2004;18(10):658–64.

21. Kenawey M, Liodakis E, Krettek C, et al. Effect of the lower limb rotational alignment on tibiofemoral contact pressure. Knee Surg Sports Traumatol Arthrosc 2011;19(11):1851–9.

22. Bretin P, O'Loughlin PF, Suero EM, et al. Influence of femoral malrotation on knee joint alignment and intra-articular contract pressures. Arch Orthop Trauma Surg 2011;131(8):1115–20.

23. Svoboda SJ, McHale K, Belkoff SM, et al. The effects of tibial malrotation on the biomechanics of the tibiotalar joint. Foot Ankle Int 2002;23(2):102–6.

24. Özbek EA, Kalem M, Kınık H. Do the Loss of Thigh Muscle Strength and Tibial Malrotation Cause Anterior Knee Pain after Tibia Intramedullary Nailing? Biomed Res Int 2019;2019:3072105.

25. Ricci WM, Bellabarba C, Lewis R, et al. Angular malalignment after intramedullary nailing of femoral shaft fractures. J Orthop Trauma 2001;15(2):90–5.

26. Patel NM, Yoon RS, Cantlon MB, et al. Intramedullary nailing of diaphyseal femur fractures secondary to gunshot wounds: predictors of postoperative malrotation. J Orthop Trauma 2014;28(12):711–4.

27. Koerner JD, Patel NM, Yoon RS, et al. Femoral malrotation after intramedullary nailing in obese versus non-obese patients. Injury 2014;45(7):1095–8.

28. Patel NM, Yoon RS, Koerner JD, et al. Timing of diaphyseal femur fracture nailing: is the difference night and day? Injury 2014;45(3):546–9.

29. Salem KH, Maier D, Keppler P, et al. Limb malalignment and functional outcome after antegrade versus retrograde intramedullary nailing in distal femoral fractures. J Trauma 2006;61(2):375–81.

30. Gardner MJ, Citak M, Kendoff D, et al. Femoral fracture malrotation caused by freehand versus navigated distal interlocking. Injury 2008;39(2):176–80.

31. Stephen DJ, Kreder HJ, Schemitsch EH, et al. Femoral intramedullary nailing: comparison of fracture-table and manual traction. a prospective, randomized study. J Bone Joint Surg Am 2002;84(9):1514–21.

32. Davids JR. Rotational deformity and remodeling after fracture of the femur in children. Clin Orthop Relat Res 1994;(302):27–35.

33. Say F, Bülbül M. Findings related to rotational malalignment in tibial fractures treated with reamed intramedullary nailing. Arch Orthop Trauma Surg 2014;134(10):1381–6.

34. Dugdale TW, Degnan GG, Turen CH. The use of computed tomographic scan to assess femoral malrotation after intramedullary nailing. A case report. Clin Orthop Relat Res 1992;(279):258–63.

35. Liodakis E, Doxastaki I, Chu K, et al. Reliability of the assessment of lower limb torsion using computed tomography: analysis of five different techniques. Skeletal Radiol 2012;41(3):305–11.

36. Kim JJ, Kim E, Kim KY. Predicting the rotationally neutral state of the femur by comparing the shape of the contralateral lesser trochanter. Orthopedics 2001;24(11):1069–70.

37. Deshmukh RG, Lou KK, Neo CB, et al. A technique to obtain correct rotational alignment during closed locked intramedullary nailing of the femur. Injury 1998;29(3):207–10.

38. Bråten M, Tveit K, Junk S, et al. The role of fluoroscopy in avoiding rotational deformity of treated femoral shaft fractures: an anatomical and clinical study. Injury 2000;31(5):311–5.

39. Clementz BG. Assessment of tibial torsion and rotational deformity with a new fluoroscopic technique. Clin Orthop Relat Res 1989;(245):199–209.

40. Clementz BG, Magnusson A. Assessment of tibial torsion employing fluoroscopy, computed tomography and the cryosectioning technique. Acta Radiol 1989;30(1):75–80.

41. Reikerås O, Høiseth A, Reigstad A, et al. Femoral neck angles: a specimen study with special regard to bilateral differences. Acta Orthop Scand 1982;53(5):775–9.

42. Langer JS, Gardner MJ, Ricci WM. The cortical step sign as a tool for assessing and correcting rotational deformity in femoral shaft fractures. J Orthop Trauma 2010;24(2):82–8.

43. Ramme AJ, Egol J, Chang G, et al. Evaluation of malrotation following intramedullary nailing in a femoral shaft fracture model: Can a 3D c-arm improve accuracy? Injury 2017;48(7):1603–8.

44. Aamodt A, Terjesen T, Eine J, et al. Femoral anteversion measured by ultrasound and CT: a comparative study. Skeletal Radiol 1995;24(2):105–9.

45. Jakob RP, Haertel M, Stüssi E. Tibial torsion calculated by computerised tomography and compared to other methods of measurement. J Bone Joint Surg Br 1980;62-B(2):238–42.

46. Stahl JP, Alt V, Kraus R, et al. Derotation of post-traumatic femoral deformities by closed intramedullary sawing. Injury 2006;37(2):145–51.

47. Mei-Dan O, McConkey MO, Bravman JT, et al. Percutaneous femoral derotational osteotomy for excessive femoral torsion. Orthopedics 2014;37(4):243–9.

48. Itoman M, Sekiguchi M, Yokoyama K, et al. Closed intramedullary osteotomy for rotational deformity after long bone fractures. Int Orthop 1996;20(6):346–9.

49. Jagernauth S, Tindall AJ, Kohli S, et al. New Technique: A Novel Femoral Derotation Osteotomy for Malrotation following Intramedullary Nailing. Case Rep Orthop 2012;2012:837325.

50. Takase K, Lee SY, Waki T, et al. Minimally Invasive Treatment for Tibial Malrotation after Locked Intramedullary Nailing. Case Rep Orthop 2018;2018:4190670.

51. Fiz N, Delgado D, Sánchez X, et al. Application of 3D technology and printing for femoral derotation osteotomy: case and technical report. Ann Transl Med 2017;5(20):400.

52. Tetsworth KD, Thorsell JD. Combined techniques for the safe correction of very large tibial rotational deformities in adults. J Limb Lengthening Reconstruction 2015;1(1):6–13.

53. Kahn KM, Beals RK. Malrotation after locked intramedullary tibial nailing: three case reports and review of the literature. J Trauma 2002;53(3):549–52.

54. van der Werken C, Marti RK. Post-traumatic rotational deformity of the lower leg. Injury 1983;15(1):38–40.

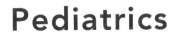

Pediatrics

Cast-Related Complications

Daniel F. Drake, MD, Todd F. Ritzman, MD*

KEYWORDS

- Cast • Complication • Decubitus • Compartment syndrome • Cast saw • Thermal injury

---

KEY POINTS

- Casting remains an important treatment modality in the armamentarium of orthopedic surgery.
- Casting is a procedure with risks and complications like any operative procedure and should be treated with the same vigilance and training.
- Optimizing casting indications, materials, technique, and removal skills are key to complication avoidance.
- Attributing patient complaints to an underlying injury or surgical field is a diagnosis of exclusion and cast-related complaints must be expediently evaluated.

INTRODUCTION

Given that techniques of external immobilization of fractures predate internal or external fixation of fractures by millennia, it is not hyperbole to state that casting is foundational to the history of orthopedic surgery. However, over the last several decades, there has been a significant and appropriate shift in emphasis to the operative reduction and fixation of fractures. With this transition, closed reduction and definitive cast treatment of extremity fractures has become less frequent yielding decreased training focus on cast application techniques, less experiential expertise in cast therapy, and less awareness of the potential complications of casting. Naturally, this care transition has contributed to the proverbial lost art of casting. However, casting continues to be an essential technique requisite for comprehensive, excellent orthopedic care; this is especially true in the subspecialty of pediatric orthopedic surgery.

CLINICAL PEARLS FOR CAST APPLICATION AND COMPLICATION AVOIDANCE

The clinical focus of this review is on complications of cast treatment and precludes a detailed discussion of cast application techniques. However, any discussion of cast complications is incomplete if it fails to address proper cast application techniques as the primary means of complication avoidance. The following concise principles are not comprehensive but should be considered for safe, effective casting:

- *Appropriate padding*: A minimum of two layers of circumferential padding applied with 50% overlap throughout cast with minimum four layers at proximal and distal junctions of cast and at bony prominences (ie, olecranon, distal humerus condyles, malleoli, heel). Excessive padding can contribute to a loose cast with inadequate immobilization of fracture reductions or joints and failure of cast therapy. Avoidance of pleating/wrinkling of cast padding is essential to avoid pressure-related symptoms on application of plaster or fiberglass cast material.
- *Appropriate thickness*: Inadequate cast material can contribute to soft or broken casts and failure of immobilization (ie, plantar breakdown of walking cast, broken first webspace bridge in upper extremity cast). Excessive cast material increases risk of thermal injury during cast removal (ie, excessively thick cast on dorsal, concave side of ankle).
- *Appropriate extremity positioning*: The individual holding the extremity during

---

Department of Orthopedic Surgery, Akron Children's Hospital, 1 Perkins Way, Akron, OH 44308, USA
* Corresponding author.
E-mail address: tritzman@akronchildrens.org

Orthop Clin N Am 52 (2021) 231–240
https://doi.org/10.1016/j.ocl.2021.03.005

cast application has an equally important role as the individual applying the cast; it is essential they understand this! Inadequate focus by the assistant can lead to joint position change and resultant wrinkling of padding or cast material at joints and impingement on soft tissue and/or bony prominences. Preprocedural instruction is imperative for the assisting provider to enable a stable platform on which to apply a cast and should be included as part of a "casting time out." Inappropriate positioning can lead to failed therapy and/or complications. The following is not a comprehensive list but serves as examples of the impact of inadequate extremity positioning. Inadequate elbow flexion can enable distal translation of a cast on a young child. Inadequate ulnar deviation of wrist/hand to avoid radial drift of distal radius fractures.[1] Hyperflexion of wrist can contribute to development of carpal tunnel syndrome. Ankle dorsiflexion in a distal one-third tibia fracture can contribute to recurvatum deformity.

- *Appropriate molding*: Casts must be molded to resist deforming forces of fractures, prevent distal translation of cast on extremity, and provide adequate joint immobilization.[2,3] "Straight casts lead to crooked bones." "Crooked casts lead to straight bones." Long arm cast: avoid the "banana cast" focusing on angular elbow position, molding straight ulnar border, interosseous mold to restore radial bow, three-point mold to maintain fracture reduction.

- *Appropriate length*: Patients and parents perceive that cast comfort and cast length are inversely proportional. At our center, the mantra is repeated that "a long arm cast is a long arm cast" and "a long leg cast is a long leg cast"; implying that casts should consistently be applied proximal on the arm or leg so as to ensure immobilization of the elbow and knee, respectively. Short casts enable significant adjacent joint motion, especially in the obese or young child with baby fat and contribute to loss of alignment in distal humerus or distal femur fractures.
  - Long arm/leg casts generally should be used for all extremity casting in children less than 2 years because short casts have propensity for distal slippage.

  - Immobilize the joint above and joint below for long bone diaphyseal or proximal metaphyseal fractures (ie, short leg cast terminating proximal to metatarsophalangeal joints for a metatarsal fracture or proximal to the toe tips for a great toe fracture, long arm cast rather than short arm cast for diaphyseal forearm fracture, hip spica cast rather than long leg cast for distal third femur fracture). In general, avoid cast treatment or modify plan to a longer cast if a cast terminates at the level of fracture.

- Avoidance of impingement on adjacent joints:
  - Excessively long casts applied with the extremity in abduction impinge in the axilla or groin once the extremity is adducted to a neutral resting position.
  - Short or long arm casts should enable functional digit use when properly applied. Cast material distal to the distal palmar flexion crease or excessive cast material over the first webspace precludes thumb and digit use during cast therapy.
  - Caution the technique of staging a short arm/leg cast to a long arm/leg cast. Impingement on the antecubital or popliteal fossa can inadvertently occur if the short cast is applied in extension and the joint is then flexed for application of the long extension (Fig. 1). Additionally, appropriate three-point and intraosseous molding is difficult, if not impossible, for the treatment of diaphyseal or proximal forearm fractures using this staged technique. Finally, inadequate overlap of the cast material when converting the short to the long leg cast can contribute to uncoupling of the two halves and failure of immobilization.

- *Appropriate duration of casting*: Inadequate cast duration can contribute to malunion, nonunion, or refracture. Excessive cast duration can lead to joint contracture and muscle atrophy and inappropriately prolong duration of disability.

- *Appropriate index of suspicion*: The phrase "there are no hypochondriacs in casts" is important to remember when evaluating a patient in a cast or splint and every effort should be made to resolve any cast-related complaint.

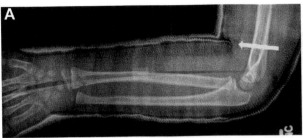 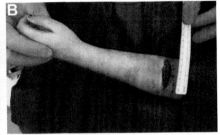

Fig. 1. (A) Radiograph demonstrating antecubital cast impingement (*arrow*). Short arm cast applied in relative elbow extension, elbow subsequently flexed to 90° and cast lengthened in staged fashion to a long arm cast. (B) Clinical photograph at time of surgical irrigation and debridement of decubitus, which ultimately required split-thickness skin graft coverage.

Attributing a focused cast complaint to the underlying injury should be considered a diagnosis of exclusion with liberal consideration for cast windowing to rule out impending decubitus (**Fig. 2**), cast univalving (**Fig. 3**) or bivalving to rule out cast compartment syndrome, or cast change.

○ High index of suspicion should be held for patients with inability to verbalize or sense cast complaints (ie, patients who are young or nonverbal, have developmental delay, head injuries, impaired cognition or prolonged sedation, patients with impaired sensation or peripheral nerve blocks).

• *Appropriate removal technique*: Thermal injuries or, less commonly, lacerations can occur during cast removal. Ensure appropriate training and expertise of all individuals using a cast saw to minimize these complications.[4]

These bullet points are intended to be generalized high-yield recommendations to facilitate successful cast treatment and avoid complications. A comprehensive discussion of indications, techniques, treatment protocols/durations, and postcasting recommendations is beyond the scope of this review. Efforts to ensure a minimum competency in orthopedic surgical training are evidenced by inclusion of casting/splinting education in the American Board of Orthopedic Surgery residency skills modules for PGY-1 residents.[5] As pediatric orthopedic surgeons, our institution has taken ownership of the responsibility of propagating the art of casting to our residents and fellows by holding an intensive bimonthly casting workshop, supporting junior residents with experienced orthopedic cast technicians in the emergency/trauma setting, and maintaining a culture of accountability and continual constructive feedback. This workshop includes didactic education, skills training for reduction and casting techniques, skills training for cast saw technique using a low-fidelity model (pool noodle) followed by progression to a human model, and final confirmation of competency before clearance.

GENERALIZED CAST COMPLICATIONS: AWARENESS AND AVOIDANCE
Skin Complications Related to Wet or Contaminated Cast

In all patients with traditional cotton cast padding, the consequences of a wet cast can contribute to underlying skin complications. At highest risk are young children or incontinent patients because it is common for a cast to become soiled with urine, feces, or other bodily fluid. Maintained moisture in a nonwaterproof (cotton-lined) cast can result in skin irritation, skin breakdown/maceration, dermatitis, cellulitis, fungal infections, and surgical site infections. A wet or soiled cast requires urgent cast removal, inspection of the underlying tissues, appropriate cleansing, and cast change. A foul-smelling cast may also be indicative of an underlying infection. The cast should be inspected fully, and windowed or removed completely to investigate the odor and inspect any underlying incision. Wound infections or cellulitis should be treated aggressively with antibiotic therapy and/or surgical irrigation and debridement. If cast changes are required frequently, other methods of fracture fixation or immobilization, such as open reduction and internal fixation or closed reduction and external fixation, should be considered. Parents should be instructed to inspect the cast intermittently and educated on proper positioning and frequent diaper changes to avoid soiling. For example, parents with children in hip spica casts are instructed on the "diaper under/diaper over" technique in which a small

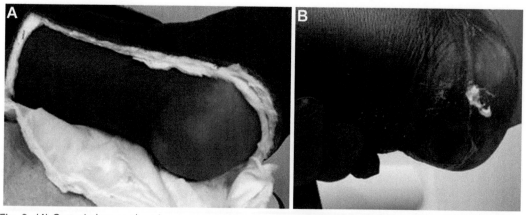

Fig. 2. (A) Cast window on short leg cast to enable evaluation of patient complaint of heel pain. (B) Follow-up photograph demonstrating development of calcaneal decubitus secondary to inadequate padding and inadequate supracalcaneal mold.

diaper is tucked under the cast and a larger diaper is more traditionally applied around the cast. Efforts to avoid cast exposure to water or fluids include the provision of "cast covers" for showering or bathing,[6,7] the use of waterproof cast liners under traditional cotton padding,[8] or the use of all-waterproof cast padding and fiberglass.[9–13] If a waterproof casting liner (ie, spica cast pantaloon) is in place with traditional cotton/fiberglass casting, cleaning under the junctions of the cast with moist cloths can often effectively avoid skin complications related to perineal soiling. The increased expense of full-waterproof casting materials is justified when considering patient satisfaction, convenience, and the ability of patients to bathe in clean, soapy water and should be considered in circumstances in which an incision or open wound does not exist under the casted extremity.

Decubitus

Decubitus are catastrophic complications of cast therapy with potential necessity of aborting cast treatment, prolonged wound therapy, and/or plastic surgical consultation.[14] A decubitus can occur if focal areas of external cast pressure exceed perfusion pressure and can occur rapidly with transient symptoms.[15] Accordingly, vigilant and expedient evaluation of patient complaints is imperative via either cast windowing or cast removal so as to identify an impending decubitus and enable revision casting, when indicated. Patient/guardian education is imperative to familiarize awareness that migration of toes or fingers in a cast predisposes to development of focal cast pressure and risk for decubitus. Concomitantly, 24-hour access must be available for casted patients/guardians to access providers to communicate concerns for cast discomfort or migration and obtain urgent evaluation. The most common location for cast-related decubitus is the heel, and the primary treatment should be avoidance via proper supracalcaneal cast molding and additional cast padding over the calcaneal tuberosity (see **Fig. 2**). Well-molded casts

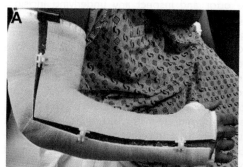
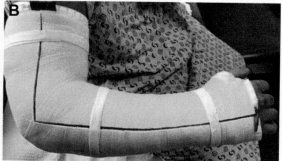

Fig. 3. (A) Long arm cast with dorsal univalve to accommodate postreduction forearm swelling. Note blue cast saw safety tape and taped cast spacers. (B) Long arm cast following removal of cast spacers and cast closure.

prevent cast migration and minimize skin shear and resultant direct contact on bony prominences. The use of additional foam padding has been shown to be an effective and inexpensive way to lower the incidence of skin complications in postoperative lower extremity casts.[16] Another risk factor for decubitus relates to retained foreign bodies in casts, which create focal areas of pressure and present additional opportunities for complications. Pen caps, rulers, coins, small toy pieces, clothes hangers and chopsticks are accidently or intentionally inserted inside a cast, often to relieve an itch leading to skin complications, which range from superficial abrasions to infected ulcerations. These complications are prevented if foreign objects are removed promptly. Additionally, in the absence of drug allergy, pruritus is relieved by submersion of a waterproof cast in warm, soapy water, hair drying a cotton or waterproof cast with the cool temperature setting, or the use of over-the-counter diphenhydramine or antihistamines.

Compartment Syndrome
Following casting, the expectation is for patients to be significantly more comfortable following immobilization of an injured extremity or fracture. Because of their circumferential nature, casts place patients at increased risk of compartment syndrome. Soft tissue swelling may increase following cast application and contribute to the development of compartment syndrome. Any patient with a cast-related complaint should be evaluated expediently. Compartment syndrome presents with the five "Ps" (increasing pain, paresthesia, pallor, paralysis, and poikilothermia) and the additional classic finding of pain with passive stretch of digits. In pediatrics, the three "As" (increased anxiety, agitation, and analgesic requirements) are assessed because patients often have difficulty or the inability to effectively communicate the pain symptoms. This should be coupled with a thorough neurovascular examination. If compartment syndrome is suspected, circumferential pressure must be relieved by univalving or bivalving with or without release of the underlying padding; evidence suggests that these maneuvers are capable of sequential decrease in intracast pressures of 40% to 65%.[17] Cast spacers or wedges may be placed to ensure the cast stays open. One experimental study demonstrates the benefit of spacing the fiberglass split by at least 6 to 9 mm (see **Fig. 3**).[18]

Thermal Injury/Cast Saw Complications
Multiple factors contribute to the risk of thermal injury either during cast application or during cast removal. The two factors most strongly associated with plaster cast–related burns include a dip water temperature greater than $50\underline{o}C$ and a cast that is too thick (>24-ply).[19,20] Plaster thickness is problematic when material is overlapped, or edges are folded over to adjust the length of splints.[21,22] Heat must be allowed to dissipate as the cast or splint sets. Studies have shown that temperatures capable of causing thermal injury are reached when casts are placed on pillows, supportive frames, or reinforced with fiberglass before allowing the materials to cure and heat to dissipate.[22] When removing casts, iatrogenic cast saw injuries occur with an incidence of 0.1% to 0.72%.[23] The "in-out technique" should be used to minimize the time the saw blade is in contact with the skin and to avoid "dragging the blade" causing abrasive injuries. Also, commercially available protective strips have been found to reduce blade-to-skin contact and reduce heat transfer when perforating casting material minimizing cast saw issues.[24] Halanski and coworkers[21,22] has thoroughly described proper cast saw technique and provides supplemental educational videos.[21,22] Other risk factors for thermal injury include the use of worn blades, fiberglass material, and casts greater than 0.5-inch thickness. Generally, ensuring cast thickness of less than three-eighths of an inch or fewer than 12 layers, appropriate thickness of underlying cast padding, and dip water temperature at room temperature is protective from thermal injury.

Joint Stiffness and Muscle Contractures
It is essential to balance the casting time required for injury and osseous union with the sequelae of disuse atrophy and joint contracture. Inadequate cast duration can contribute to malunion, nonunion, or refracture necessitating revision treatment or alteration in treatment. Excessive cast duration can lead to joint contracture and muscle atrophy, and inappropriately prolong duration of disability. Additionally, when feasible, there are opportunities to safely shorten the duration of casting or avoid cast treatment altogether via the use of removable splints or pneumatic walking boots.[25] For example, when treating torus fractures of the distal radius and ulna, review suggests nonrigid immobilization methods have advantages over rigid cast immobilization, including lower

complication rate, lower treatment cost, earlier return of function, and higher satisfaction.[26–28]

Disuse Osteopenia and Adjacent Pathologic Fractures

The length of time a patient is placed in cast immobilization must be carefully considered to prevent or limit unwanted physiologic changes. More functional casts (patellar tendon-bearing cast) or bracing alternatives (ie, pneumatic walking boot) may help increase a patient's extremity motion and decrease the length of time needed for cast treatment, thereby minimizing unwanted physiologic changes and the risks associated with cast treatment. Patients with paralytic conditions, cerebral palsy, and those taking anticonvulsant medications likely experience further disuse osteopenia with immobilization. This further increases the patient's risk for pathologic fracture during the casting period and on cast removal. Whenever feasible, cast duration should be limited to 4 weeks to help avoid a downward spiral of immobilization and worsening disuse osteopenia.

Delayed Diagnosis of Wound Infections

Most patients placed in postsurgical casts heal without incident. However, when casts are covering wounds, incisions or pins, the diagnosis of a wound infection has the potential to be delayed. Unexplained fever, increased pain at the surgical site, drainage from the cast, and/or foul smell all warrant a thorough examination of the cast with windowing or removal to assess the underlying wound. Physicians and patients must be aware that severe infectious complications, although uncommon, is associated with cast and splint treatment.[29] Cases of toxic shock syndrome and necrotizing fasciitis have been described. These patients must undergo appropriate medical work-up and surgical irrigation and debridement.

COMPLICATIONS ASSOCIATED WITH SPECIFIC CAST TYPES

Hip Spica Cast

Hip spica cast treatment is recommended for diaphyseal femur fractures in patients age 6 months to 5 years of age with less than 2 cm of fracture shortening.[30] Thus, appropriate patient selection and treatment indications are critical to minimize hip spica cast complications. Patients at either extreme of age (<6 months, >5 years) or with fractures with excessive shortening (>2 cm) should be considered for alternative treatment. Infantile patients less than 6 months of age are treated with Pavlik

harness therapy with excellent results and avoidance of cast-related complications.[31] Older patients (>5 yr) or patients with excessive fracture shortening (>2 cm) have a higher likelihood of malunion or complications in hip spica cast treatment and could be considered for alternative surgical therapy, such as flexible intramedullary nailing or submuscular plating.[32,33] Volkmann contracture and compartment syndrome are rare complications associated with hip spica cast treatment of pediatric femur fractures.[34] In Mubarak and coworkers'[34] published series, all patients were treated with 90/90 spica casts in which an initially applied below knee cast was used to position the extremity and apply traction while the remainder of the spica cast was applied. On shortening of the fracture in the cast, all children developed skin and deep muscular necrosis of the proximal, posterior calf and seven of nine patients had anterior ankle decubitus with full-thickness skin loss (**Fig. 4**). The authors recommend avoiding 90/90 hip and knee flexion in preference for a 45° angle of flexion of both joints, avoidance of applying the extremity cast first in preference for a proximal to distal cast application technique, and leaving the ipsilateral foot uncasted with a supramalleolar stopping point (**Fig. 5**). Hip spica casts have marked propensity for perineal soiling of urine or feces and have significant associated incidence of dermal complications and skin excoriation with occasional requirement for unplanned cast change in the operating room. Waterproof pantaloon liners or waterproof padding have been used with significant decrease in the incidence of skin excoriation with resultant decrease in need for unplanned hip spica cast changes (skin complications decreased from 22% decreased to 1%, unplanned cast change decreased from 14% to 3%).[8]

Cotton Versus Waterproof Cast

The complications related to a wet or soiled cast can largely be avoided with use of waterproof casting materials. Except for extremities on which open, traumatic, or surgical wounds exist or in which percutaneous pins are present, waterproof cast padding overwrapped with fiberglass cast material is used without compromising clinical outcome.[11] Waterproof casts have been shown to be equivalent to traditional casting in maintenance of alignment with the benefit of improved patient satisfaction and decreased skin irritation, odor, pruritus, and need for cast changes.[8,12,13] Verbal and written instructions must be available to patients/

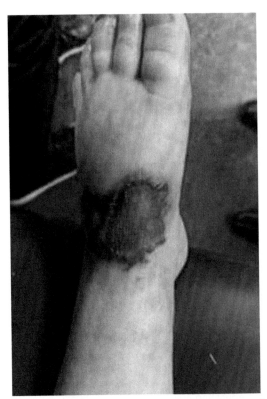

Fig. 4. Dorsal foot decubitus related to shortening of femur fracture in hip spica cast in which foot was included in initially applied long leg cast.

guardians receiving waterproof cast materials. Specifically, casts can be fully submerged in clean or chlorinated water; contaminated lake or saltwater should be avoided because

entrapped debris, sand, or salt is a skin irritant; and patients should avoid freezing outdoor temperatures for several hours after a cast is wet. Waterproof cast materials are more expensive than traditional cotton cast padding; however, when considering the benefit to the patient, cost savings of decreased frequency of unplanned cast changes, and decrease in skin-related complications, many practitioners or institutions easily justify this cost difference.

Clubfoot Cast

Serial Ponseti casting for gradual correction of clubfoot deformity carries a unique complication profile given the recurring nature of casting, intentionally thin cast padding use to enable sequential molding, and challenges unique to treating awake infants. Plaster remains the preferred casting material for Ponseti casting because of its moldability and ease of removal, although most high-volume centers remove casts with a cast saw, plaster casts are soaked and removed if difficulty or discomfort is encountered. Dip water temperature should not exceed room temperature and plaster ply thickness should not exceed 12 or the patient is at risk for thermal injury during the exothermic reaction of plaster curing. Semirigid "soft cast" material has also been shown to have equivalent efficacy to traditional plaster in Ponseti casting with the benefit of cast saw avoidance by simple unwrapping for removal.[35,36] The challenges of casting an awake infant are addressed by environmental influences, such as ambient light,

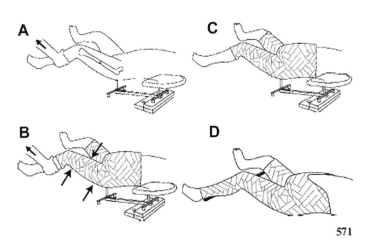

Fig. 5. Authors' recommended technique of spica cast application. (A) The patient is placed on a child's fracture spica table. The leg is held in about 45° angle of flexion at the hip and knee with traction applied to the proximal calf. (B) The 1.5 spica is then applied down to the proximal calf. Molding of the thigh is accomplished during this phase. (C) Radiographs of the femur are obtained and any wedging of the cast that is necessary can occur at this point in time. (D) The leg portion of the cast and the cross bar are applied. The belly portion of the spica is trimmed to the umbilicus. (From Mubarak, S., Frick, S., Sink, E., Rathjen, K. and Noonan, K., 2006. Volkmann Contracture and Compartment Syndromes after Femur Fractures in Children Treated with 90/90 Spica Casts. *Journal of Pediatric Orthopaedics*, 26(5), pp.567-572; with permission)

571

soothing music, suckling or pacifier use, and a specialized, high-volume team.

Postsurgical/Post-traumatic Cast

At our institution, it is common practice to immediately cast surgical and post-traumatic patients with liberal use of immediate cast univalving and 1-cm spacer application to accommodate swelling. This practice may be controversial because many centers use noncircumferential splints in the immediate postinjury or postsurgical setting with outpatient overwrap or change to circumferential casting once swelling has dissipated. Patient anxiety and office efficiency are optimized with this practice of immediate casting because patients avoid the discomfort of a cast change at early follow-up and avoid the cumbersome size and bulky appearance of a fiberglass overwrapped splint. Additionally, surgeon and cast technician workflow are not interrupted with the need to hold, cast, and mold the extremity at the time of splint change. Additionally, in scenarios in which radiographic surveillance is not required, guardians are instructed to untape, remove, close, and retape a cast while at home 1-week postapplication enabling avoidance of unnecessary follow up appointments; this proves a convenience for families and outpatient office access (see **Fig. 3**).

SUMMARY

Despite the advances in surgical techniques and technology, casting remains an important treatment modality in the armamentarium of orthopedic surgery. However, because of those advances in techniques and technology, opportunities for skill development and complication management are a decreasing commodity for the surgeon in training. Although the exact incidence of complications is unknown, significant morbidity may be associated with a cast complication when it presents and may have medicolegal implications. The most common cast complications include a wet or soiled cast, thermal and cast saw injuries, decubitus, joint stiffness/contractures, compartment syndrome, and disuse osteopenia/adjacent pathologic fractures. Every effort should be made to urgently resolve a patient with a cast or splint-related complaint. Knowing the potential complications associated with casts and splints, preventative techniques and how to counsel patients and caregivers appropriately help provide safe and high-quality care with minimal complications. Given that nonoperative management via casting remains a significant portion of the pediatric

orthopedic surgeon's practice, it is imperative that pediatric orthopedic training centers remain vigilant at teaching safe, efficacious casting techniques so as to avoid fulfillment of the proverbial lost art of casting for future generations of surgeons. Following the lead of the American Board of Orthopedic Surgery Resident Skills Modules, we implore teaching institutions to develop and maintain robust teaching programs, skills acquisitions laboratories, and assessments for confirmation of competency for all residency programs.[4,37–39]

CLINICS CARE POINTS

- Casting is a procedure with risks just like any operative procedure; treat it as such. These risks are best avoided with preparation, sound decision making, and technical expertise. A preprocedure casting time-out should be performed identifying patient, identifying extremity, confirming availability and preparation of materials to ensure efficient cast application, and introducing and educating assisting roles of all involved teammates.

- Never change joint position once cast padding or fiberglass is applied. Doing so risks wrinkling of cast material and impingement.

- "A long arm is a long arm cast. A long leg cast is a long leg cast." Do not stop short on arm or thigh because, despite patient perception, a shorter cast permits more motion, contributes to more pain, and potentially converts a nondisplaced fracture to a displaced fracture.

- Caution in the antecubital fossa/popliteal fossa when converting short arm cast to long arm cast or short leg cast to long leg cast. The short cast, if applied in extension, impinges in fossa when flexed into desired joint position risking soft tissue impingement, decubitus, or compartment syndrome.

- Optimize the team's proficiency and safety at cast removal. Use protective cast removal strips. Avoid overly thick casts. Ensure the use of sharp blades. Check blade temperature and cool blades frequently. Develop training processes or workshops for surgeons in training, advanced practice providers, and orthopedic cast technicians before direct patient care.

- "There is no such thing as a hypochondriac in a cast!" Attributing cast complaints to the underlying injury or surgical field is a diagnosis of exclusion. Cast windows should be used freely or casts should be removed to enable inspection of bony prominences, open wounds, surgical incisions, and so forth. Patients must have direct access to care and evaluation for cast concerns 24/7 because decubitus, compartment syndrome, and other complications can develop rapidly. When in doubt, rapidly progress through the continuum of univalve, bivalve, removal of half of cast, or removal of entire cast.

DISCLOSURE

The authors have nothing to disclose.

REFERENCES

1. Edmonds EW, Capelo RM, Stearns P, et al. Predicting initial treatment failure of fiberglass casts in pediatric distal radius fractures: utility of the second-metacarpal-radius angle. J Child Orthop 2009; 35(5):375–81.
2. Wenger DR, Pring ME, Rang M. Rang's children's fractures. 3rd edition. Philadelphia: Lippincott Williams & Wilkins; 2005.
3. Sarmiento A, Latta L. Functional fracture bracing: tibia, humerus and ulna. New York: Springer; 1995.
4. Bae DS, Lynch H, Jamieson K, et al. Improved safety and cost savings from reductions in cast-saw burns after simulation-based education for orthopaedic surgery residents. J Bone Joint Surg 2017;99(1–6):e94.
5. Parsons BO, Jeffries JT. Module#5 casting techniques: splints, casts, and removal. In: ABOS residency skills modules for PGY-1 residents. Available at: https://www.abos.org/wp-content/uploads/2019/07/Module-5-Casting-Techniques-Splints-Casts-and-Removal.pdf. Accessed January 15, 2020.
6. McDowell M, Nguyen S, Schlechter J. A comparison of various contemporary methods to prevent a wet cast. J Bone Joint Surg Am 2014;96:e99.
7. Nielsen DM, Ribley LG, Ricketts DM. Keeping plaster casts dry: what works? Injury 2005;36:73–4.
8. Wolff CR, James P. The prevention of skin excoriation under children's hip spica casts using the Goretex Pantaloon. J Pediatr Orthop 1995;15:386–8.
9. Stevenson AW, Gahukamble AD, Antoniou G, et al. Waterproof cast liners in pediatric forearm fractures: a randomized trial. J Child Orthop 2013;7:123–30.
10. Guillen PT, Fuller CB, Riedel BB, et al. A prospective randomized crossover study on the comparison of cotton versus waterproof cast liners. Hand 2016;11:50–3.
11. Robert CE, Jiang JJ, Khoury JG. A prospective study on the effectiveness of cotton versus waterproof cast padding in maintaining the reduction of pediatric distal forearm fractures. J Pediatr Orthop 2011;31:144–9.
12. Shannon EG, DiFazio R, Kasser J, et al. Waterproof casts for immobilization of children's fractures and sprains. J Pediatr Orthop 2005;25:56–9.
13. Haley CA, DeJong ES, Ward JA, et al. Waterproof versus cotton cast liners: a randomized, prospective comparison. Am J Orthop 2006;35:137–40.
14. Lee TG, Chung S, Chung YK. A retrospective review of iatrogenic skin and soft tissue injuries. Arch Plast Surg 2012;39(4):412–6.
15. Halanski M, Noonan KJ. Cast and splint immobilization: complications. J Am Acad Orthop Surg 2008;16:30–40.
16. Murgai RR, Compton E, Patel AR, et al. Foam padding in postoperative lower extremity casting: an inexpensive way to protect patients. J Pediatr Orthop 2018;38(3):e470–4.
17. Garfin SR, Mubarak SJ, Evans KL, et al. Quantification of intracompartmental pressure and volume under plaster casts. J Bone Joint Surg Am 1981; 63(3):449–53.
18. Kleis K, Schlechter JA, Doan JD, et al. Under pressure: the utility of spacers in univalved fiberglass casts. J Pediatr Orthop 2019;39(6):302–5.
19. Gannaway JK, Hunter JR. Thermal effects of casting materials. Clin Orthop Relat Res 1983;181:191–5.
20. Lavalette R, Pope MH, Dickstein H. Setting temperatures of plaster casts: the influence of technical variables. J Bone Joint Surg Am 1982;64: 907–11.
21. Halanski MA. How to avoid cast saw complications. J Pediatr Orthop 2016;36:S1–5.
22. Halanski MA, Halanski AD, Oza A, et al. Thermal injury with contemporary cast-application techniques and methods to circumvent morbidity. J Bone Joint Surg Am 2007;89:2369–77.
23. Ansari MZ, Swarup S, Ghani R, et al. Oscillating saw injuries during removal of plaster. Eur J Emerg Med 1998;5:37–9.
24. Stork NC, Lenhart RL, Nemeth BA, et al. To cast, to saw, and not to injure: can safety strips decrease cast saw injuries? Clin Orthop Relat Res 2016; 474(7):1543–52.
25. Shirley ED, Maguire KJ, Mantica AL, et al. Alternatives to traditional cast immobilization in pediatric patients. J Am Acad Orthop Surg 2020;28:e20–7.
26. Kuba MH, Izuka BH, Feese KP. One visit-one brace: patient and parent satisfaction after treatment for pediatric distal radius buckle fractures. J Pediatr Orthop 2017;37:157.
27. Neal E. Comparison of splinting and casting in the management of torus fracture. Emerg Nurse 2014; 21:22–6.

28. Boutis K, Howard A, Constantine E, et al. Evidence into practice: pediatric orthopaedic surgeon use of removable splints for common pediatric fractures. J Pediatr Orthop 2015;35:18–23.

29. Delasobera BE, Place R, Howell J, et al. Serious infectious complications related to extremity cast/splint placement in children. J Emerg Med 2011;41(1):47–50.

30. Roaten JD, Kelly DM, Yellin JL, et al. Pediatric femoral shaft fractures: a multicenter review of the AAOS clinical practice guidelines before and after 2009. J Pediatr Orthop 2019;39(8):394–9.

31. Podeszwa DA, Mooney JF, Cramer KE, et al. Comparison of Pavlik harness application and immediate spica casting for femur fractures in infants. J Pediatr Orthop 2004;24:460–2.

32. Assaghir Y. The safety of titanium elastic nailing in preschool femur fractures: a retrospective comparative study with spica cast. J Pediatr Orthop B 2013; 22:289–95.

33. Heffernan MJ, Gordon JE, Sabatini CS, et al. Treatment of femur fractures I young children: a multicenter comparison of flexible intramedullary nails to spica casting in young children aged 2-6 years. J Pediatr Orthop 2015;35:126–9.

34. Mubarak SJ, Frick S, Sink E, et al. Volkmann contracture and compartment syndromes after femur fractures in children treated with 90/90 spica casts. J Pediatr Orthop 2006;26:567–72.

35. Aydin BK, Sofu H, Senaran H, et al. Treatment of clubfoot with Ponseti method using semirigid synthetic softcast. Medicine 2015;94:e2072.

36. Hui C, Joughin E, Nettel-Aguirre A, et al. Comparison of cast materials for the treatment of congenital idiopathic clubfoot using the Ponseti method: a prospective randomized controlled trial. Can J Surg 2014;57:247–53.

37. Difazio RL, Harris M, Feldman L, et al. Reducing the incidence of cast-related skin complications in children treated with cast immobilization. J Pediatr Orthop 2017;37(8):526–31.

38. Balch Samora J, Samora WP, Dolan K, et al. A quality improvement initiative reduces cast complications in a pediatric hospital. J Pediatr Orthop 2018;38(2):e43–9.

39. Shore BJ, Hutchinson S, Harris M, et al. Epidemiology and prevention of cast saw injuries: results of a quality improvement program at a single institution. J Bone Joint Surg Am 2014;96(4):e31.

Hand and Wrist

Common Complications of Distal Radial Fractures

Hayden S. Holbrook, MD*, Travis A. Doering, MD, Benjamin M. Mauck, MD

KEYWORDS

- Distal radial fractures • Treatment • Complications • Avoiding complications
- Treating complications

KEY POINTS

- Outcomes of distal radial fractures generally are good; however, complications have been reported in up to 30% of operatively treated fractures.
- Potential complications can be associated with each treatment strategy, operative and nonoperative, as well as with specific fracture patterns and patient-specific factors.
- Complications may involve the bones, joints, soft tissues, tendons, and nerves.
- The risk of complications can be decreased by careful preoperative planning and meticulous surgical technique.
- Complications should be recognized and treated promptly to avoid poor outcomes.

Distal radial fractures (DRF) are one of the most common fractures treated by orthopedic surgeons. In 1998, more than 640,000 DRFs were reported in the United States alone.[1] In a separate 2009 epidemiologic study, a bimodal distribution of DRF was demonstrated to exist in those under 18 years and over 65 years (30.18 and 25.42 per 10,000 person-years, respectively).[2] The incidence of DRF continues to increase as both the worldwide life expectancy and the rate of osteoporosis increases. Nonoperative management with immobilization, as well as multiple operative fixation strategies, are used for the treatment of DRF. These operative techniques may include some combination of external fixation, percutaneous pinning, intramedullary fixation, or plate fixation. Although the treatment outcomes of DRF are generally good, studies have reported complication rates between 8% and 27% in operatively treated DRF.[3–7] A knowledge of the potential complications associated with each treatment strategy, as well as with specific fracture patterns, will help to prevent complications before they occur and recognize and treat complications when they do occur.

Before beginning a treatment course with a patient with a DRF, it is imperative to obtain a thorough history and perform a thorough physical examination to assess the patient's preinjury activity level, demands placed on the injured extremity, and support network, in addition to any nerve, tendon, or concomitant injuries to be better able to discuss the patient's desired goals and predicted outcomes once treatment is completed. Presenting the potential known adverse outcomes of a specific treatment strategy also is critical and helps to maintain the patient's trust when complications do arise. This review describes common complications that are encountered when treating a DRF, ways to prevent complications, and how to recognize and treat complications when they do occur.

OSSEOUS COMPLICATIONS

Malunion

Although recorded treatment of DRF exists within Egyptian-era case reports dating back approximately 5000 years ago,[8] it was not until Abraham Colles's publication in 1814 that our modern understanding of DRF began.[9]

Department of Orthopaedic Surgery & Biomedical Engineering, University of Tennessee-Campbell Clinic, Memphis, TN, USA
* Corresponding author. 1211 Union Avenue, Suite 500, Memphis, TN 38104.
E-mail address: hholbro2@uthsc.edu

Orthop Clin N Am 52 (2021) 241–250
https://doi.org/10.1016/j.ocl.2021.03.009

Conservative management with a wooden splint was standard treatment until 1895, when Wilhelm Röntgen published his Nobel Prize winning work on x-rays.[10] Although this advance would pave the way for more sophisticated treatment of DRF in the future, it also allowed an immediate assessment of fracture patterns and the position in which nonoperatively treatment fractures healed. The resulting identification of loss of radial height, radial inclination, and volar tilt are the common deformities that continue to occur with closed reduction and cast immobilization of extra-articular fractures today. Additionally, radiographs allowed for the identification of intra-articular fractures and subsequent incongruities of the articular surface.

Significant debate still exists on the optimal treatment of DRF, particularly for displaced fractures in the physiologically elderly population. Because malunion remains the most common complication after nonoperative management ($\leq$24% in historical series), several high-quality randomized controlled trials have recently attempted to answer this question, without clear answer.[11] The American Academy of Orthopedic Surgeons published clinical practice guidelines suggesting that a postreduction dorsal tilt of more than 10°, radial shortening of more than 3 mm, or intra-articular displacement of more than 2 mm indicates the need for a discussion regarding the benefits of surgical fixation.[12] Although many malunions that fall outside these criteria are asymptomatic, it has been shown that at 2 years in general patients with malunion have higher pain scores and lower levels of function.[13,14] Several authors have attempted to identify patient-specific and fracture-specific findings that may lead to a subsequent loss of reduction and healing in a malunited state, such as the LeFontaine criteria, but not all of these criteria have been reproduced in subsequent studies.[15,16] Biomechanically, the alternation of distal radial geometry can affect the function of the upper extremity in several ways, which are discussed along with treatment in subsequent sections: articular incongruity can lead to post-traumatic arthritis, shortening of the distal radius leads to relative lengthening and increased load on the ulna, and dorsal tilt leads to sigmoid notch impingement and carpal malalignment.

Ulnar styloid fractures commonly occur in conjunction with DRF. It is estimated that 53% of DRFs have an associated ulnar styloid fracture and 26% of these go on to nonunion.[17] This fracture pattern has raised concerns among orthopedic surgeons in that this concomitant injury may lead to instability of the distal radioulnar joint (DRUJ) and ulnar-sided wrist pain. Multiple studies have shown that there is no difference in function or outcome in patients with DRF with associated ulnar styloid fractures treated with volar plating.[18–20] Studies have also demonstrated that the healing status (ie, the presence of persistent ulnar styloid nonunion) of the ulnar styloid does not affect outcomes.[18,21] Ozasa and colleagues[22] demonstrated that the presence of an ulnar styloid nonunion does not have an adverse effect on outcomes after osteotomy correction of a distal radial malunion. If the DRUJ is found to be unstable by examination after the completion of fixation of the DRF, the ulnar styloid fracture should be treated with open reduction and internal fixation with repair of the triangular fibrocartilage complex, when indicated. The DRUJ of the uninjured wrist should be carefully examined and compared with the injured wrist before surgery.

Sigmoid Notch Impingement

The sigmoid notch makes up the ulnar side of the distal radius that articulates with the distal ulna, together forming the DRUJ. The sigmoid notch is a concave or flat surface, covered with articular cartilage, that provides stability to the DRUJ and allows protonation and supination of the forearm. Sigmoid notch impingement can be the result of intra-articular displacement of fractures involving the sigmoid notch, displacement of an extra-articular DRF with radial translation or shortening, or iatrogenic screw breach into the DRUJ. Intra-articular extension-type DRFs have been estimated to involve the sigmoid notch in 76% of DRFs based on computed tomography evaluation.[23] Failure to correct the displacement of the sigmoid notch can lead to a decreased range of motion, arthrosis, and pain. Acceptable limits of articular step-off of the sigmoid notch have not been described, although most apply evidence for radiocarpal joint step-off.[24,25]

Radial translation or coronal shift of the distal radial articular segment occurs with some DRFs. This pattern can cause sigmoid notch impingement and ultimately DRUJ instability. Anatomic studies have pointed toward the distal oblique bundle as 1 source of this instability. The distal oblique bundle runs obliquely from the ulna proximally to the radius distally and is one of many stabilizing structures of the DRUJ. With radial translation of the distal radius, the distal oblique bundle becomes slack and the stabilizing function of this structure is lost.[26]

Radial shortening, a common deformity found in DRFs, alters the relationship of the ulnar head within the sigmoid notch, predisposing to impingement. The radioulnar contact area is shifted proximally to a point of less articular congruence.[27] Altered DRUJ biomechanics can present with limited forearm rotation. Radial shortening also leads to ulnar impaction, which is discussed in the section on Ulnar Impingement. Ultimately, an incongruent DRUJ can be the result of a disruption of the articular surface by a fracture line within the sigmoid notch, extra-articular deformity (radial translation or radial shortening) of the distal radius affecting the DRUJ joint surface, or a combined mechanism.

Last, iatrogenic screw penetration through the sigmoid notch can lead to pain and rapid arthrosis of the DRUJ. Fixation of volar ulnar corner fractures poses the greatest risk of screw breach. Capturing of this fracture fragment with screws within the intermediate column is especially important for carpal stability and is discussed in greater detail elsewhere in this article. It is difficult to assess the articular reduction or screw penetration into the DRUJ with intraoperative fluoroscopy because of the shape of the sigmoid notch.[28] The modified skyline view of the sigmoid notch can be obtained with the wrist in extension and 10° to 15° of dorsal angulation to the x-ray beam.[29] This positioning allows a perpendicular view of the sigmoid notch to detect articular step-off. The sunrise view and the extended tangential view have also been described as means to identify screw breach into the sigmoid notch.[30] In general, penetration of the DRUJ with a screw is due to either to a nonanatomic reduction or improper plate placement.

The treatment of sigmoid notch impingement is challenging, particularly in a healed fracture. Although a computed tomography scan through the DRUJ with the wrist in neutral, pronation, and supination can be helpful, a clinical assessment of pronosupination before definitive treatment may be a more applicable method of assessment. If identified before healing, open reduction and internal fixation with a careful intraoperative assessment of forearm rotation is the treatment of choice. If identified after the sigmoid notch has healed in a malunited position with limitation of motion, a sigmoid notch reconstruction with osteotomy, reduction, and fixation of the volar lunate facet is indicated.

Ulnar Impingement

The relative ulnar length is commonly affected by a DRF. Ulnar variance is defined as the change in length of the ulna relative to the length of the distal radius. Normally, the radius and ulna are approximately the same length and this is best viewed on a true posterior to anterior radiographic view of the wrist with the shoulder abducted to 90°. Small changes in the relative length of the ulna to the radius lead to changes in force transmission through the carpus. Biomechanical testing has shown that 84% of the axial load through the hand is transmitted through the radius and 16% is transferred through the triangular fibrocartilage complex disc and ulnar column.[31] Subsequent biomechanical studies demonstrated that lengthening of the ulna by 2.5 mm (ulnar positive) increased force transmission through the ulna to 41.9% and shortening of the ulna by 2.5 mm (ulnar negative) decreased axial load through the ulna to 4.3%.[31] DRFs are commonly associated with concomitant relative lengthening of the ulna (ulnar positive), resulting in ulnar impaction on the ulnar carpus while simultaneously affecting the DRUJ, as described previously. Repetitive abutment of the ulnar carpus by the distal ulna results in degenerative changes to the triangular fibrocartilage complex, lunate, and triquetrum.

The implications of ulnar variance for functional outcomes of patients with distal radial malunions has been studied. A prospective study of 123 patients who had closed reduction and casting, percutaneous pinning, or external fixation of DRFs showed worse Disability of the Arm, Shoulder, and Hand (DASH) scores at 2 years in patients with distal radial malunions with ulnar variance of 1 mm or more.[14] A retrospective study of 297 conservatively treated DRFs with an average of 3.5-year follow-up showed unsatisfactory results in 42% of patients with more than 5 mm of relative ulnar lengthening.[32]

Distal radial osteotomies and ulnar shortening osteotomies have been described to manage distal radial malunions with ulnar impaction with the goal of neutralizing ulnar variance. Distal radial osteotomies for ulnar abutment are more technically challenging and have more complications, longer operative times, and typically require additional procedures for bone graft harvesting.[33] Osteotomies for DRF malunions can be approached via a volar, dorsal, or anterolateral approach, but given the usefulness of volar locking plating, most malunions can be corrected with an opening wedge osteotomy from a volar approach. The choice of bone graft affects outcomes.[34]

Lunate Escape

Intra-articular DRFs can result in a number of characteristic fracture patterns that are based on the injury mechanism and ligamentous attachments.[35,36] Studies have called attention to the volar lunate facet fragment as a source of fixation failure and lunate escape if not recognized and managed appropriately.[37] The volar lunate facet fragment is the origin of the short radiolunate ligament, and the loss of its integrity can lead to volar displacement, or lunate escape, of the carpus. Given the normal anatomy of the distal radius volar cortex, sloping volarly from radial to ulnar, standard volar plates may be unsuccessful at supporting both the scaphoid and lunate facets.[37] Harness and colleagues[37] reported 7 patients who lost fixation of the volar lunate facet resulting in carpal subluxation; 5 required revision fixation. The teardrop angle, the angle subtended by the central portion of the tear drop and the radial shaft, has been used to assess the lunate facet in intra-articular fractures on the 10° tilt lateral radiograph.[38,39] The narrow width and rapid transition to the volar surface of the lunate facet make plate fixation and screw purchase difficult within this fragment.[40] Fixation of this fragment is important both for the support of the carpus and stabilization of the DRUJ because it involves sigmoid notch.

Multiple fixation options exist for the volar lunate facet. External fixation combined with plating of the volar lunate facet, headless compression screws, and Kirschner wire fixation techniques have been described to support the volar ulnar corner fragment.[41–43] Newer implants have been designed specifically with this challenging fracture pattern in mind. The volar hook plate uses 2 tines that are placed through predrilled extra-articular slots into the lunate facet.[44,45] As the hook plate is placed distal to the watershed line, surgeons should consider elective implant removal owing to flexor tendon concerns, although this concern is minimized with newer low-profile plates. Alternative fixation techniques should be considered with fragments less than 5 mm.[45] A critical analysis of the preoperative imaging will help to choose an appropriate implant when treating this complex fracture pattern and prevent volar escape of the carpus.

Carpal Malalignment

Carpal malalignment is defined as displacement on a lateral view of the longitudinal axis of the capitate either dorsally or volarly to the longitudinal axis of the radius. The dorsal subluxation is thought to be secondary to the loss of palmar tilt of the articular surface of the distal radius in malunited DRFs.[46] The carpus adapts to the dorsal deformity of the distal radius with flexion through the midcarpal joint or with extension in a volar deformity.[47] This particular form of carpal instability nondissociative—dorsal intercalary segment instability (CIND-DISI) has been shown to decrease grip and pinch strength at 1 year.[48] Recognizing carpal malalignment is critical both when deciding whether fracture alignment is acceptable for conservative treatment and when assessing an intraoperative reduction. Malalignment can be identified easily on a lateral radiograph when the longitudinal axis of the capitate and radius intersect outside of the carpus or when the center of the proximal pole of the capitate fails to reside within a rectangle drawn from the volar and dorsal cortex of the radius.[49] Malunited fractures with dorsal tilt of more than 10° and ulnar variance of more than 1 mm have been shown to have lower scores on the DASH questionnaire at 2 years.[14] Failure to correct carpal malalignment of DRFs requires osteotomy for correction of malunited fractures in symptomatic patients.

SOFT TISSUE COMPLICATIONS

Acute Carpal Tunnel Syndrome

Acute carpal tunnel syndrome (ACTS) can occur secondary to trauma to the distal radius or other traumatic injuries to the wrist or hand and is less common than carpal tunnel syndrome. Unlike carpal tunnel syndrome, ACTS requires urgent surgical intervention to prevent complications. ACTS presents with pain and dysesthesias in the median nerve distribution in the hand owing to an acute rise in pressure within the carpal tunnel and can be contrasted with carpal tunnel syndrome owing to its acute temporal presentation.[50] ACTS is rapid in onset and progressive over a course of hours. With ACTS, the compartmental pressure of the carpal tunnel exceeds the epineural blood supply to the median nerve leading to ischemia and ultimately pain and dysesthesias. DRFs are the most common cause of ACTS.[51] Risk factors for ACTS after DRF include a high-energy mechanism of injury and fracture translation.[52] Volar displacement of fracture fragments of the distal radius causing stretch of the median nerve, direct contact of fracture fragments against the median nerve, and hematoma development can lead to ACTS or median nerve contusion. Differentiating between the two is critical given their differing treatments. Median nerve contusion presents with immediate sensory loss, whereas patients with ACTS initially present with normal sensation that progresses to a loss in 2-point discrimination.[53] This finding highlights the importance of serial examinations in diagnosing ACTS. A median nerve contusion is monitored expectantly with rest and observation, in contrast with ACTS.

Treatment of ACTS is surgical decompression, although simultaneous treatment of the associated DRF requires thoughtful preoperative planning. Surgical decompression is urgent and better results have been shown in patients who had surgical release before 40 hours. In 1 study, 4 of 5 patients released before 40 hours had regained full sensation within 96 hours after surgery. An additional 3 patients with ACTS who were released at 6, 9, and 33 days showed incomplete recovery at 3 months or longer.[53] Carpal tunnel release can be performed through a single incision combined with an extended flexor carpi radialis approach or a 2-incision approach with a traditional longitudinal palmar incision and separate trans–flexor carpi radialis or volar Henry approach. In a prospective cohort of 27 patients with DRFs without ACTS, the extended flexor carpi radialis approach was demonstrated to be safe and effective for the treatment of the concurrent DRF when compared with a single volar Henry approach.[54] Proponents of the 2-incision technique have raised concerns of injury to the palmar cutaneous sensory branch of the median nerve along the ulnar side of the flexor carpi radialis tendon sheath during the single-incision approach.

Tendon Injury

The flexor and extensor tendons are at risk with both operative and nonoperative treatment of DRFs as they glide across the volar and dorsal cortex. Tendon issues may present as painful tenosynovitis or frank tendon rupture.

With the nonoperative treatment of DRFs, rupture of the extensor pollicis longus (EPL) tendon has been described. It is thought that the risk of EPL rupture is greater with nondisplaced or minimally displaced DRFs as a result of a competent extensor retinaculum in these lower energy fracture patterns.[55] A retrospective review estimated the rate of EPL rupture in 61 nondisplaced fractures as 5%.[56] This complication was recognized at an average of 6.6 weeks after injury. Direct repair often is untenable owing to attritional rupture, and so a tendon transfer using the extensor indicis proprius or another donor often is required.

Percutaneous pinning with Kirschner wires for the treatment of DRF places the flexor and extensor tendons, as well other anatomic structures, at risk. Percutaneous pinning can be used for temporary intraoperative reduction, for definitive fixation in isolation, or in combination with other fixation constructs for the treatment of the distal radius. When used, Kirschner wires are most commonly placed through the radial styloid, the dorsal rim distal to Lister's tubercle, or a transverse subchondral wire buttressing an intra-articular fracture.[57] The anatomic study by Chia and colleagues[57] offered recommendations of pin placement based on cadaver dissections. The radial styloid and transverse radial pin placed the superficial branch of the radial nerve and the abductor pollicis longus tendon at risk. The dorsal wire should be placed within 5 mm of the ulnar side of Lister's tubercle to protect the extensor digitorum communis, while simultaneously avoiding the EPL coursing around Lister's tubercle. They recommend a 1- to 2-cm incision be made before pin placement to avoid tendon or nerve injury.

Bridge plating has been indicated for unstable comminuted fractures, osteoporotic fractures in patients requiring early weight bearing, significant soft tissue injuries, and dorsal shear patterns.[4] Bridge plating can be used in isolation or in conjunction with volar plating or percutaneous fixation. Distally, the bridge plate is fixed to either the second or third metacarpal. Plating to the third metacarpal has a greater risk of entrapping the EPL tendon and the tendons of the first dorsal compartment and displaces the extensor digitorum communis tendons.[58] Plating to the second metacarpal places branches of the superficial radial nerve at risk when approaching the metacarpal. Hanel and colleagues[59] analyzed complications with dorsal bridge plating in 144 fractures and reported 1 case of EPL rupture and 2 cases of digital stiffness requiring tenolysis. They also reported implant failure, infection, malunion, and nonunion. Their overall complication rate decreased from 20.8% to 8.5% in patients who had their plates removed before 16 weeks, suggesting early plate removal as a means to decrease complications, although this finding was not statistically significant.[59]

Volar locked plating has become one of the most common methods for the operative treatment of DRFs. As the use of volar locked plating has increased, associated complications with its use have become apparent. Complications associated with implants have been cited as the most common adverse event.[5] The relationship of the flexor tendons to the most volar prominence of the distal radius, or the watershed line, places them at risk. Soong and colleagues[7] introduced a classification system that depends on the position of the volar locking plate. This grading scheme is based on the relationship of the volar plate to a line drawn through the volar tip of the distal radius parallel to the radial shaft on a lateral radiograph, referred to as the critical line. Distal plating to the watershed line brings the plate in closer contact with the traversing flexor tendons placing them at risk for attritional rupture and pressure necrosis.[60,61] Flexor tendons are put at risk both by distal plating volar to the critical line and with thicker volar plates, both of which are exacerbated by insufficient restoration of volar tilt. Tendons may be abraded by the volar plate or by prominent screw heads with repetitive movement. Symptomatic implants may present as a painful tenosynovitis of the flexor tendons or a complete rupture of a flexor tendon.[62] FPL tendon and index finger flexor digitorum profundus tendon ruptures have been reported.[63] Application of the Soong classification has shown higher rates of implant removal of plates sitting distal and volar to the watershed line.[64] Some have recommended plate removal after fracture union in symptomatic patients with plates sitting 2 mm volar to the critical line.[61] As with an EPL rupture, attrition of the FPL or FDP tendons makes primary repair challenging, and so tendon transfer using FDS of the ring finger or other donor is often necessary.

On the dorsal surface of the distal radius, screw prominence becomes a source of extensor tendon complications when using volar locked plates. Screws of improper length may protrude from the dorsal cortex of the distal radius and impinge on the traversing extensor tendons. With time, repetitive microtrauma of the extensor tendons against penetrating screw tips leads to painful tendon irritation, tenosynovitis, and eventual attritional tendon rupture. The anatomy of the dorsal distal radius, specifically the prominence of Lister's tubercle, makes standard intraoperative lateral fluoroscopic imaging difficult to identify screw penetration. On lateral and protonation views of the distal radius, a prominent dorsal screw is masked by the cortical shadow of Lister's tubercle.[65] The dorsal tangential view or skyline view is obtained by flexing the elbow to approximately 70°, supinating the forearm, and fully flexing the wrist. Adjustments in elbow flexion and extension are performed until an optimal view is obtained with Lister's tubercle at its maximal height and the radial styloid and dorsal ulnar corner are visible.[65,66] When dorsal screw penetration is identified on the dorsal tangential view, the

screw can be exchanged for one of a shorter length to minimize the risk of extensor tendon irritation. Similarly, some surgeons advocate using unicortical locking screws in the distal segment to entirely eliminate the risk of screw irritation. Biomechanical studies have shown 75% unicortical screw lengths have a similar stability and construct stiffness to bicortical fixation.[67,68]

Surgical Site Infection

Infections after DRF fixation are uncommon and may be associated with the presence of an open fracture, treatment method, age, and patient sex.[69] A large, country-wide database identified a rate of infection of 5% after open reduction with plate fixation, 12% after percutaneous pinning, and 28% after external fixation. Published rates of surgical site infections in case series range from 3% to 5% across all operatively managed DRFs, but are increased in the presence of several patient or fracture related factors. Smoking (odds ratio, 3.79), presence of a Kirschner wire/external fixator (odds ratio, 3.73), and uncontrolled diabetes mellitus (hemoglobin A1c >7; odds ratio, 7.83) are some of the strongest predictors of postoperative infection. The evidence is mixed for infection rates after surgical treatment of open DRFs; some studies show no increased risk for Gustillo 1 or 2 fractures, even with elective or delayed management,[70,71] whereas other studies have shown increased rates of infection for contaminated Gustillo 2/3 or Swanson 2 open fractures despite multiple initial debridements.[72] Another key finding across these studies is that it did not seem that the time to initial debridement influenced infection rates. The management of surgical site infections with oral antibiotics alone was sufficient for most cases, although more complex or contaminated injuries occasionally required more aggressive interventions, including irrigation and debridement, implant removal, and occasionally conversion to a wrist fusion.

Complex Regional Pain Syndrome

Complex regional pain syndrome (CRPS) complicates the recovery of patients after operatively and nonoperatively treated DRFs, and is a challenging complication for both the patient and the provider. CRPS syndrome is composed of chronic pain, autonomic dysfunction, trophic changes, and hand dysfunction.[73] Commonly, patients with DRFs present with warmth, edema, stiffness, shiny skin, and pain refractory to narcotics. The prevalence has been reported in 2 of 1000 patients with DRF and an incidence of 0.64%.[74,75] CRPS type 1 is the more common type after DRF management, because type 2 CRPS occurs as an inappropriate pain response after an injury to a specific nerve. Risk factors include older age, female sex, open fractures, associated distal ulnar fractures, and rheumatoid arthritis.[74,75] There also is a strong association with coexisting diagnosis of fibromyalgia.[74,76] Surgeon-dependent risk factors for CRPS include excessive cast tightness in nonoperatively treated fractures and overdistraction of the carpus with external fixation or dorsal bridge plating in operatively treated fractures.[77]

Vitamin C has been studied as a pharmacologic aid to decrease the incidence of CRPS. Its mechanism of action is thought to interfere with the toxic free radical inflammatory response mediated by oxygen. Two separate studies by Zollinger and colleagues[78,79] demonstrated a significant reduction in CRPS with a daily dose of 500 mg vitamin C. These 2 studies were limited by their subjective diagnosis of CRPS. Despite these drawbacks, the results from this group led the American Academy of Orthopedic Surgery to recommend the use of vitamin C for the prevention of CRPS in 2010.[12] A more recent prospective, double-blinded, randomized controlled trial of 336 patients showed no benefit of vitamin C in decreasing the incidence of CRPS or improvement in DASH score and raised concerns for the efficacy of vitamin C for preventing CRPS.[80]

Much of the diagnosis of CRPS depends on the physical examination—an inspection of the hand for swelling, posturing, moisture, or dryness; palpation for hyperalgesia; motor and sensory examination; and range of motion of joints. Additional diagnostic testing includes pain thresholds with dolorimeters, autonomic dysfunction testing, 3-phase bone scans, and sympatholytic challenge testing.[39] Early diagnosis and treatment for CRPS are recommended. Treatment typically combines hand therapy with pharmacologic aids. Hand therapy includes passive and active range of motion exercises, splinting, and alternating warm and cool baths. Pharmacologic options with sympatholytic components include antidepressants, anticonvulsants, membrane-stabilizing agents, and adrenergic agents.

SUMMARY

Overall, the treatment of DRF is associated with reliably good outcomes; however, although they occur at low rates, complications can significantly impair the success of treatment. Therefore, the treating surgeon should be fully aware of potential complications associated with each treatment type and how to best prevent them. Although certain patient-specific and fracture-specific factors may increase the risk of adverse outcomes, most are nonmodifiable risk factors at the time of presentation and so it is imperative that every effort is made to mitigate these risk factors to prevent long-term morbidity. Additionally, patients should be well-informed about these complications and potential symptoms so that they may be address expeditiously.

DISCLOSURE

Neither the authors nor their immediate family received any financial payments or other benefits from any commercial entity related to the subject of this article.

REFERENCES

1. Chung KC, Spilson SV. The frequency and epidemiology of hand and forearm fractures in the United States. J Hand Surg 2001;26(5):908–15.
2. Karl JW, Olson PR, Rosenwasser MP. The epidemiology of upper extremity fractures in the United States, 2009. J Orthop Trauma 2015; 29(8):e242–4.
3. Arora R, Lutz M, Hennerbichler A, et al. Complications following internal fixation of unstable distal radius fracture with a palmar locking-plate. J Orthop Trauma 2007;21(5):316–22.
4. Lauder A, Hanel DP. Spanning bridge plate fixation of distal radial fractures. JBJS Rev 2017;5(2). 01874474-201702000-00002.
5. Pidgeon TS, Casey P, Baumgartner RE, et al. Complications of volar locked plating of distal radius fractures: a prospective investigation of modern techniques. Hand (N Y) 2020;15(5):698–706.
6. Rozental TD, Blazar PE. Functional outcome and complications after volar plating for dorsally displaced, unstable fractures of the distal radius. J Hand Surg 2006;31(3):359–65.
7. Soong M, van Leerdam R, Guitton TG, et al. Fracture of the distal radius: risk factors for complications after locked volar plate fixation. J Hand Surg 2011;36(1):3–9.
8. Breasted JH. The Edwin Smith surgical papyrus. Special ed. Birmingham (AL): The Classics of Medicine Library; 1984.
9. Colles A. On the fracture of the carpal extremity on the radius. Edinb Med Surg J 1814;10:182–6.
10. Rontgen WC. On a new kind of rays. Ober eine neue Art von Strahlen. In: Sitzungsberichte der Wurzburger Physik.-Medic.- Gesellschaft. 1895.

11. Katt B, Seigerman D, Lutsky K, et al. Distal radius malunion. J Hand Surg 2020;45(5):433–42.

12. Lichtman DM, Bindra RR, Boyer MI, et al. Treatment of distal radius fractures. J Am Acad Orthop Surg 2010;18(3):180–9.

13. Ali M, Brogren E, Wagner P, et al. Association between distal radial fracture malunion and patient-reported activity limitations: a long-term follow-up. J Bone Joint Surg Am 2018;100(8):633–9.

14. Brogren E, Wagner P, Petranek M, et al. Distal radius malunion increases risk of persistent disability 2 years after fracture: a prospective cohort study. Clin Orthop Relat Res 2013;471(5): 1691–7.

15. Lafontaine M, Hardy D, Delince P. Stability assessment of distal radius fractures. Injury 1989;20(4): 208–10.

16. Walenkamp MM, Aydin S, Mulders MA, et al. Predictors of unstable distal radius fractures: a systematic review and meta-analysis. J Hand Surg Eur Vol 2016;41(5):501–15.

17. Bacorn RW, Kurtzke JF. Colles' fracture; a study of two thousand cases from the New York State Workmen's Compensation Board. J Bone Joint Surg Am 1953;35-a(3):643–58.

18. Sammer DM, Shah HM, Shauver MJ, et al. The effect of ulnar styloid fractures on patient-rated outcomes after volar locking plating of distal radius fractures. J Hand Surg 2009;34(9):1595–602.

19. Souer JS, Ring D, Matschke S, et al. Effect of an unrepaired fracture of the ulnar styloid base on outcome after plate-and-screw fixation of a distal radial fracture. J Bone Joint Surg Am 2009;91(4): 830–8.

20. Zenke Y, Sakai A, Oshige T, et al. The effect of an associated ulnar styloid fracture on the outcome after fixation of a fracture of the distal radius. J Bone Joint Surg Br 2009;91(1):102–7.

21. Buijze GA, Ring D. Clinical impact of united versus nonunited fractures of the proximal half of the ulnar styloid following volar plate fixation of the distal radius. J Hand Surg 2010;35(2):223–7.

22. Ozasa Y, Iba K, Oki G, et al. Nonunion of the ulnar styloid associated with distal radius malunion. J Hand Surg 2013;38(3):526–31.

23. Tanabe K, Nakajima T, Sogo E, et al. Intra-articular fractures of the distal radius evaluated by computed tomography. J Hand Surg 2011;36(11): 1798–803.

24. Knirk JL, Jupiter JB. Intra-articular fractures of the distal end of the radius in young adults. J Bone Joint Surg Am 1986;68(5):647–59.

25. Missakian ML, Cooney WP, Amadio PC, et al. Open reduction and internal fixation for distal radius fractures. J Hand Surg 1992;17(4):745–55.

26. Dy CJ, Jang E, Taylor SA, et al. The impact of coronal alignment on distal radioulnar joint stability following distal radius fracture. J Hand Surg 2014; 39(7):1264–72.

27. Xing SG, Chen YR, Xie RG, et al. In vivo contact characteristics of distal radioulnar joint with malunited distal radius during wrist motion. J Hand Surg 2015;40(11):2243–8.

28. Kamal RN, Leversedge F, Ruch DS, et al. The sigmoid notch view for distal radius fractures. J Hand Surg 2018;43(11):1038.e1–5.

29. Klammer G, Dietrich M, Farshad M, et al. Intraoperative imaging of the distal radioulnar joint using a modified skyline view. J Hand Surg 2012;37(3): 503–8.

30. Klein J, Mijares M, Chen D, et al. Radiographic evaluation of the distal radioulnar joint: technique to detect sigmoid notch intra-articular screw breach in distal radius fractures. Tech Orthop 2018;35:1.

31. Palmer AK, Werner FW. Biomechanics of the distal radioulnar joint. Clin Orthop Relat Res 1984;187: 26–35.

32. Altissimi M, Antenucci R, Fiacca C, et al. Long-term results of conservative treatment of fractures of the distal radius. Clin Orthop Relat Res 1986;(206): 202–10.

33. Aibinder WR, Izadpanah A, Elhassan BT. Ulnar shortening versus distal radius corrective osteotomy in the management of ulnar impaction after distal radius malunion. Hand (N Y) 2018;13(2): 194–201.

34. Ring D, Roberge C, Morgan T, et al. Osteotomy for malunited fractures of the distal radius: a comparison of structural and nonstructural autogenous bone grafts. J Hand Surg Am 2002;27:216–22.

35. Mandziak DG, Watts AC, Bain GI. Ligament contribution to patterns of articular fractures of the distal radius. J Hand Surg 2011;36(10):1621–5.

36. Rhee PC, Medoff RJ, Shin AY. Complex distal radius fractures: an anatomic algorithm for surgical management. J Am Acad Orthop Surg 2017;25(2): 77–88.

37. Harness NG, Jupiter JB, Orbay JL, et al. Loss of fixation of the volar lunate facet fragment in fractures of the distal part of the radius. J Bone Joint Surg Am 2004;86(9):1900–8.

38. Fujitani R, Omokawa S, Iida A, et al. Reliability and clinical importance of teardrop angle measurement in intra-articular distal radius fracture. J Hand Surg 2012;37(3):454–9.

39. Medoff RJ. Essential radiographic evaluation for distal radius fractures. Hand Clin 2005;21(3):279–88.

40. Andermahr J, Lozano-Calderon S, Trafton T, et al. The volar extension of the lunate facet of the distal radius: a quantitative anatomic study. J Hand Surg 2006;31(6):892–5.

41. Moore AM, Dennison DG. Distal radius fractures and the volar lunate facet fragment: Kirschner

wire fixation in addition to volar-locked plating. Hand (N Y) 2014;9(2):230–6.

42. Ruch DS, Yang C, Smith BP. Results of palmar plating of the lunate facet combined with external fixation for the treatment of high-energy compression fractures of the distal radius. J Orthop Trauma 2004;18(1):28–33.

43. Waters MJ, Ruchelsman DE, Belsky MR, et al. Headless bone screw fixation for combined volar lunate facet distal radius fracture and capitate fracture: case report. J Hand Surg 2014;39(8):1489–93.

44. Bakker AJ, Shin AY. Fragment-specific volar hook plate for volar marginal rim fractures. Tech Hand Up Extrem Surg 2014;18(1):56–60.

45. O'Shaughnessy MA, Shin AY, Kakar S. Volar marginal rim fracture fixation with volar fragment-specific hook plate fixation. J Hand Surg 2015; 40(8):1563–70.

46. Taleisnik J, Watson HK. Midcarpal instability caused by malunited fractures of the distal radius. J Hand Surg 1984;9(3):350–7.

47. Ng CY, McQueen MM. What are the radiological predictors of functional outcome following fractures of the distal radius? J Bone Joint Surg Br 2011;93(2):145–50.

48. McQueen MM, Hajducka C, Court-Brown CM. Redisplaced unstable fractures of the distal radius: a prospective randomised comparison of four methods of treatment. J Bone Joint Surg Br 1996; 78(3):404–9.

49. Wolfe SW. Distal radius fractures. In: Wolfe SW, Hotchkiss RN, Pederson WC, et al, editors. Green's operative hand surgery. 7th edition. Elsevier, Inc; 2017. p. 516–87.

50. Schnetzler KA. Acute carpal tunnel syndrome. J Am Acad Orthop Surg 2008;16(5):276–82.

51. Bauman TD, Gelberman RH, Mubarak SJ, et al. The acute carpal tunnel syndrome. Clin Orthop Relat Res 1981;(156):151–6.

52. Dyer G, Lozano-Calderon S, Gannon C, et al. Predictors of acute carpal tunnel syndrome associated with fracture of the distal radius. J Hand Surg 2008; 33(8):1309–13.

53. Mack GR, McPherson SA, Lutz RB. Acute median neuropathy after wrist trauma. The role of emergent carpal tunnel release. Clin Orthop Relat Res 1994;300:141–6.

54. Tannan SC, Pappou IP, Gwathmey FW, et al. The extended flexor carpi radialis approach for concurrent carpal tunnel release and volar plate osteosynthesis for distal radius fracture. J Hand Surg 2015; 40(10):2026–31.e1.

55. Helal B, Chen SC, Iwegbu G. Rupture of the extensor pollicis longus tendon in undisplaced Colles' type of fracture. Hand 1982;14(1):41–7.

56. Roth KM, Blazar PE, Earp BE, et al. Incidence of extensor pollicis longus tendon rupture after nondisplaced distal radius fractures. J Hand Surg 2012;37(5):942–7.

57. Chia B, Catalano LW 3rd, Glickel SZ, et al. Percutaneous pinning of distal radius fractures: an anatomic study demonstrating the proximity of K-wires to structures at risk. J Hand Surg 2009;34(6): 1014–20.

58. Lewis S, Mostofi A, Stevanovic M, et al. Risk of tendon entrapment under a dorsal bridge plate in a distal radius fracture model. J Hand Surg 2015; 40(3):500–4.

59. Hanel DP, Ruhlman SD, Katolik LI, et al. Complications associated with distraction plate fixation of wrist fractures. Hand Clin 2010;26(2):237–43.

60. Agnew SP, Ljungquist KL, Huang JI. Danger zones for flexor tendons in volar plating of distal radius fractures. J Hand Surg 2015;40(6):1102–5.

61. Kitay A, Swanstrom M, Schreiber JJ, et al. Volar plate position and flexor tendon rupture following distal radius fracture fixation. J Hand Surg 2013; 38(6):1091–6.

62. Snoddy MC, An TJ, Hooe BS, et al. Incidence and reasons for hardware removal following operative fixation of distal radius fractures. J Hand Surg 2015;40(3):505–7.

63. Soong M, Earp BE, Bishop G, et al. Volar locking plate implant prominence and flexor tendon rupture. J Bone Joint Surg Am 2011;93(4):328–35.

64. Selles CA, Reerds STH, Roukema G, et al. Relationship between plate removal and Soong grading following surgery for fractured distal radius. J Hand Surg Eur Vol 2018;43(2):137–41.

65. Ozer K, Toker S. Dorsal abegential view of the wrist to detect screw penetration to the dorsal cortex of the distal radius after volar fixed-angle plating. Hand (N Y) 2011;6(2):190–3.

66. Vaiss L, Ichihara S, Hendriks S, et al. The utility of the fluoroscopic skyline view during volar locking plate fixation of distal radius fractures. J Wrist Surg 2014;3(4):245–9.

67. Baumbach SF, Synek A, Traxler H, et al. The influence of distal screw length on the primary stability of volar plate osteosynthesis–a biomechanical study. J Orthop Surg Res 2015;10:139.

68. Wall LB, Brodt MD, Silva MJ, et al. The effects of screw length on stability of simulated osteoporotic distal radius fractures fixed with volar locking plates. J Hand Surg 2012;37(3):446–53.

69. Rudgren J, Enocson A, Järnbert-Pettersson H, et al. Surgical site infections after distal radius fracture surgery: a nation-wide cohort study of 31,807 adult patients. BMC Musculoskelet Disord 2020;21:845.

70. Kurylo JC, Axelrad TW, Tornetta P 3rd, et al. Open fractures of the distal radius: the effects of delayed debridement and immediate internal fixation on infection rates and the need for secondary procedures. J Hand Surg Am 2011;36(7):1131–4.

71. Henry TW, Matzon JL, McEntee RM, et al. Outcomes of type I open distal radius fractures: a comparison of delayed and urgent open reduction internal fixation. Hand (N Y) 2020. https://doi.org/10.1177/1558944720964965. 1558944720964965.

72. Glueck DA, Charoglu CP, Lawton JN. Factors associated with infection following open distal radius fractures. Hand (N Y) 2009;4(3):330–4.

73. Li Z, Smith BP, Tuohy C, et al. Complex regional pain syndrome after hand surgery. Hand Clin 2010;26(2):281–9.

74. Crijns TJ, van der Gronde B, Ring D, et al. Complex regional pain syndrome after distal radius fracture is uncommon and is often associated with fibromyalgia. Clin Orthop Relat Res 2018;476(4):744–50.

75. Jo YH, Kim K, Lee BG, et al. Incidence of and risk factors for complex regional pain syndrome type 1 after surgery for distal radius fractures: a population-based study. Sci Rep 2019;9(1):4871.

76. Lipman MD, Hess DE, Werner BC, et al. Fibromyalgia as a predictor of complex regional pain syndrome after distal radius fracture. Hand (N Y) 2019;14(4):516–22.

77. Biyani A. Over-distraction of the radio-carpal and mid-carpal joints following external fixation of comminuted distal radial fractures. J Hand Surg 1993;18(4):506–10.

78. Zollinger PE, Tuinebreijer WE, Breederveld RS, et al. Can vitamin C prevent complex regional pain syndrome in patients with wrist fractures? A randomized, controlled, multicenter dose-response study. J Bone Joint Surg Am 2007;89(7):1424–31.

79. Zollinger PE, Tuinebreijer WE, Kreis RW, et al. Effect of vitamin C on frequency of reflex sympathetic dystrophy in wrist fractures: a randomised trial. Lancet 1999;354(9195):2025–8.

80. Ekrol I, Duckworth AD, Ralston SH, et al. The influence of vitamin C on the outcome of distal radial fractures: a double-blind, randomized controlled trial. J Bone Joint Surg Am 2014;96(17):1451–9.

Complications of Volar Plating of Distal Radial Fractures: A Review

Norfleet B. Thompson, MD

KEYWORDS

• Distal radial fractures • Volar plating • Complications • Avoiding complications

KEY POINTS

• Volar plating is a frequently used method of fixation of distal radial fractures, with generally good results.
• Complications can occur from injury to nerves, vessels, bones, and joints.
• The risk of implant-related complications can be decreased by careful preoperative planning and meticulous surgical technique.
• Complications may require further surgery, such as nerve or tendon repair, arthrodesis, or arthroplasty.

Distal radial fractures represent the most common upper extremity fracture treated in emergency departments. US data from 2009 show an incidence of 16.2 distal radius fractures per 10,000 persons, equating to more than 530,000 distal radius fractures.[1] The economic cost of these injuries amounts to more than US$480 million annually with US$170 million publicly funded through Medicare.[2] Patients of all ages are affected in a bimodal distribution, with young patients sustaining high-energy injuries and elderly patients susceptible to low-energy osteoporotic fractures.[3]

A variety of methods exist to treat distal radial fractures. Compared with nonoperative treatment with closed reduction and casting and other methods of stabilization (Kirschner wires, external fixation, intramedullary fixation, dorsal bridge plating), volar plating has become increasingly used, especially among younger surgeons.[4] Volar plate fixation allows biomechanically stable reduction of most distal radial fractures, facilitating early range of motion and good functional outcomes. The increasing use of this treatment method necessitates a thorough understanding of the possible complications of its use. A recent systematic review estimated a 15% overall complication rate and 5% major complication rate associated with volar plating of distal radial fractures.[5] Surgeons should be knowledgeable about these potential complications to help patients through the process of informed consent, to prevent complications when possible, and to treat adverse events in a timely manner when they do occur. Complications of volar plating have been categorized in several ways: by chronology (immediate, early, and late), by severity (major or minor), by frequency, and by type (nerve, tendon, bone, implant).[5–9]

NERVE COMPLICATIONS

Carpal tunnel syndrome is the most common complication associated with volar plating of distal radial fractures. The condition exists in 3% to 4% of the population at baseline, and it may increase to an incidence of 7% to 15% after distal radial fractures regardless of treatment.[5] With volar plate fixation, the rate of postoperative carpal tunnel syndrome generally is cited as 2% to 5%,[10,11] with rates at high as 17%.

Department of Orthopaedic Surgery & Biomedical Engineering, University of Tennessee-Campbell Clinic, 1211 Union Avenue, Suite 500, Memphis, TN 38104, USA
E-mail address: nbthompson@campbellclinic.com

Orthop Clin N Am 52 (2021) 251–256
https://doi.org/10.1016/j.ocl.2021.03.010
0030-5898/21/© 2021 Elsevier Inc. All rights reserved.

Although the position and placement of a volar plate itself may theoretically affect median nerve function in the distal forearm, other factors likely play a more significant role, including swelling from the fracture hematoma, nerve contusion from fracture displacement, errant retractor placement during surgery, or residual fracture angulation and callus affecting the nerve. Prophylactic carpal tunnel release at the time of volar plate application may be indicated for severe median nerve dysfunction on preoperative examination. Likewise, an early postoperative carpal tunnel release is reasonable for worsening symptoms. Many patients can be managed expectantly for mild paresthesias that are improving, reserving a delayed carpal tunnel release for persistently symptomatic patients. A retrospective review of 576 cases of volar plate fixation of distal radial fractures by Thorninger and colleagues[12] in 2017 reported carpal tunnel release in 2.6% of patients.

Although the median nerve is the most commonly affected nerve after volar plating, injury to other nerves may occur. In less than 1% of cases, paresthesias or neuropathy may be identified in the distributions of the palmar cutaneous branch of the median nerve, the superficial radial nerve, or the ulnar nerve.[10,13] The palmar cutaneous branch of the median nerve is particularly susceptible to iatrogenic injury during the standard volar approach through the tendon sheath of the flexor carpi radialis tendon. Complex regional pain syndrome (CRPS) is typically reported at an incidence of less than 3%, but has been reported as high as 9%.[6,9,10] More common in women, this debilitating condition is identified by disproportionate pain; sensitivity to touch; stiffness; and various vasomotor, sudomotor, and trophic changes. In the past, CRPS type 1 was distinguished from CRPS type 2 by the presence of nerve injury in type 2. More recently, the Budapest criteria have assisted in diagnosis.[14] CRPS should be recognized early and treated with a multidisciplinary approach. Standard treatment combines physical and occupational therapists with pain management specialists. Psychological and behavioral health assistance may be required. Carpal tunnel release can potentially benefit these patients with CRPS type 2.[15] The usefulness of vitamin C (typically 500 mg by mouth daily for 6–8 weeks) as a preventive strategy is based on low-quality and controversial studies. In conclusion, Alter and colleagues,[5] in a systematic review of complications of distal radial fractures, identified an overall rate of 5.7% for nerve dysfunction. Careful surgical

dissection and accurate placement of retractors and implants minimizes the risk of these injuries, whereas early recognition and prompt treatment may mitigate the effects of established nerve injury.

TENDON COMPLICATIONS

After nerve dysfunction, tendon complications are the second most common complications resulting from volar plating of distal radial fractures. The overall tendon complication rates generally vary between 1% and 3%.[7,9,10,16,17] Tendinopathy is more common than complete rupture; however, complete rupture of either extensor or flexor tendons may occur. The extensor pollicus longus is the most common extensor tendon to rupture, and the flexor pollicus longus (FPL) is the most commonly ruptured flexor tendon.[18] The recent study by Thorninger and colleagues[12] of 576 distal radial fractures reported an extensor tendon rupture rate of 2% and flexor tendon rupture rate of 0.9%.

Tendon rupture may result from an acute laceration on sharp fracture fragments or, more commonly, from attritional rupture associated with tendon irritation over regions of comminuted bone. Drill bits may injure tendons acutely during plate and screw placement, and prominent hardware can lead to delayed tendon rupture. Extensor tendons are at risk by screws penetrating the dorsal cortex of the radius. On the volar side, loose screws may back out, leading to flexor tendon irritation. In systematic review, Alter and colleagues[5,6] showed that screw loosening and screw prominence are rare, with a rate of 0.13% and 0.05%, respectively. Plate placement has received special attention since Soong and colleagues[17] established a grading system for assessing the prominence of the volar plate on the distal radius. The Soong grades 0, 1, and 2 categorize the plate position in relation to the so-called critical line (a line tangential to the volar rim and parallel to the volar cortex of the radial shaft) and the volar rim. Plate position within the critical line and proximal to the volar rim is graded Soong 0. Plate position extending volar to the critical line but still proximal to the volar rim is graded Soong 1. Plate position both volar to the critical line and at or beyond the volar rim is graded Soong 2. Although there is controversy regarding a strict relationship between Soong grade and flexor tendon complications, it is advisable to avoid plate prominence in the watershed region. Selles and colleagues[19] showed a rate of plate removal 6 times higher with volar plates with Soong grade 2 prominence. Certain plate designs may have higher or lower risk of flexor tendon irritation. In the original Soong and colleagues[17] study, the Acumed Acu-Loc plate was associated with a 4% flexor tendon rupture rate with 2 of 3 cases associated with Soong grade 2 position, whereas the Depuy DVR plate was not associated with flexor tendon rupture. Newer-generation plates are designed to minimize the risk of tendon irritation. When fracture configuration requires very distal placement of the plate or the use of specific juxta-articular or volar rim plates, it has been suggested to plan plate removal after fracture healing at 3 months.[16] Clinical symptoms and signs suggestive of tendinopathy include increasing pain at the volar wrist and crepitus or discomfort with pressure of the volar wrist as the patient flexes and extends the fingers. Tendinopathy may lead to tendon rupture within a few months of surgery or in a delayed fashion even several years later.[20] One study found FPL rupture occurred at an average of 10 months postoperatively.[21]

Surgeons should take preventive measures to avoid flexor and extensor tendon complications. Careful surgical exposure combined with accurate placement of plate and screw constructs is paramount. In general, screws in the distal flare of a volar plate need not be longer that 75% of the anterior-posterior diameter of the distal radius to secure fracture stability.[9,22] Avoiding penetration of the dorsal cortex protects vulnerable extensor tendons. Placement of the plate beyond the volar rim and volar to the critical line should be avoided unless necessary for fracture stability. Special fluoroscopic views, including the skyline view and a 23° lateral view, can reduce the risk of dorsal screw prominence and intra-articular screw penetration, respectively. The skyline view, described by Vaiss and colleagues,[23] can be obtained with the forearm supinated, elbow flexed to 75°, and the wrist completely flexed with small adjustments as directed by fluoroscopy.

IMPLANT COMPLICATIONS

Problems related to implants constitute the third category of complications of volar plating, with an incidence of 1.6% in systematic reviews by Alter and colleagues.[5,6] As stated previously, poorly placed volar plates or loosening screws may impinge on flexor tendons. Screw prominence at the dorsal cortex or screw penetration into the radiocarpal or distal radioulnar joint (DRUJ) may occur, resulting in extensor tendon injury, painful range of motion, and posttraumatic arthritis. Breakage of modern plates is rare but should raise concern for infection, nonunion, and loss of reduction. Loss of reduction itself may be considered an implant complication. Quadlbauer and colleagues[8] noted an incidence of 2% for loss of reduction with volar plating in a retrospective review of 392 cases. Even though volar plating has emerged as a popular treatment option for treatment of displaced distal radial fractures, surgeons should be aware of fracture patterns at high risk of failure with volar plating. Distal fracture fragments involving the volar ulnar corner of the distal radius predispose to subsequent volar displacement of the carpus with escape of this fragment over the end of the plate. Surgeons should be cognizant of the multiple strategies available to address this concern, including the use of a juxta-articular or volar rim plates (designed intentionally for distal fixation with planned removal after bony union), specialized hook extensions on newer-generation plates, and supplemental fixation with a dorsal bridge plate, external fixator, or radiocarpal pin. Dorsal ulnar corner fractures, dorsal shear fractures, and impacted articular fragments also may require alternative fixation or supplemental fixation in addition to volar plating. Radial styloid fractures can be treated with radial column plates or Kirschner wires/headless compression screws for simpler styloid fractures. In addition, severely comminuted fractures may not be appropriate for volar plating alone. In the retrospective review by Quadlbauer and colleagues,[8] 73% of all complications occurred in Arbeitsgemeinschaft für Osteosynthesefragen (AO) type C fractures with AO type C3 fractures accounting for 53% of all complications. To minimize implant complications, it is essential that surgeons both carefully select and appropriately apply an implant for the particular fracture being treated and use supplemental fixation if needed. Planned or unplanned removal of implants may be necessary. A recent systematic review reported overall implant removal incidence varying from 0% to 26%, and 2 recent retrospective studies showed overall implant removal rates close to 6%.[7,24]

BONE AND JOINT COMPLICATIONS

The best attempts at volar plate fixation of distal radial fractures do not prevent all complications involving the bone and joint. Malunion, delayed union, and nonunion may all occur. Although definitions vary, American Academy of

Orthopaedic Surgeons' Appropriate Use Criteria define inadequate reduction as greater than 3-mm radial shortening, greater than 10° dorsal tilt, and/or greater than 2-mm articular step-off. Delayed union can be defined as incomplete healing at 3 to 4 months, and nonunion defined as incomplete healing at 6 months requiring revision surgery with bone grafting.[7,10] Early loss of fixation from inadequate stabilization or infection leads to malunion if left untreated, and later loss of fixation suggests delayed union or nonunion. Alter and colleagues[5,6] found a malunion rate of 0.61%, but malunion requiring revision occurred in only 0.05% of patients. Lee and colleagues,[10] in a retrospective review of 1921 patients undergoing volar plate fixation, found a delayed union rate of 0.26% and a nonunion rate of 0.15%. Malunion should be treated with revision surgery after discussion with the patient, whereas delayed union can be observed while medical optimization for fracture healing is undertaken. Symptomatic nonunion requires revision fixation with possible bone graft or possibly partial or total wrist arthrodesis.

Posttraumatic osteoarthritis and stiffness are additional complications related to the bone and joint. Malunion, unidentified intra-articular screw penetration, and extrinsic and/or intrinsic carpal ligamentous injury associated with distal radial fracture predispose to posttraumatic arthritis. Posttraumatic osteoarthritis was reported in less than 1% of patients in several recent articles,[7,25,26] but was distinguished from malunion and loss of fixation. Ulnar-sided wrist pain from DRUJ incongruity, DRUJ instability, or ulnar impaction should also be considered a complication of volar plating in certain cases. DRUJ stability should be assessed with shuck testing intraoperatively during volar plate fixation and treated with splinting, DRUJ pinning, or (rarely) fixation of a large ulnar styloid fragment or triangular fibrocartilage complex injury. When nonoperative treatments fail, persistently symptomatic osteoarthritis after volar plating can be treated with partial or total wrist fusion or arthroplasty. Ulnar impaction may require ulnar shortening, and DRUJ arthritis may be considered for an open or arthroscopic wafer procedure, matched hemiresection or implant arthroplasty, or Darrach procedure in low-demand patients. In general, arthrofibrosis with severely limited motion is rare after volar plating. Bony radioulnar synostosis preventing forearm rotation has been reported in only 0.03% of patients.[5,6] However, patients should be counseled that some loss of terminal flexion and extension and forearm rotation is expected.

One study found steady improvements in range of motion for 12 months before plateauing at a reported arc of 87% flexion, 90% extension, 94% pronation, and 99% supination versus control wrist.[27]

OTHER COMPLICATIONS

In very rare cases, volar plating of distal radial fractures may lead to other serious complications, including vascular injury, compartment syndrome, and infection. Radial injury requiring repair has been reported as 0.5% overall, with the risk skewed slightly toward AO C-type fracture.[7] A crossing branch of the radial artery is often encountered in the distal portion of the extended volar flexor carpi radialis surgical approach; this branch can be safely cauterized or tied off. The radial artery proper is located in close proximity to the brachioradialis tendon and should be carefully protected. Compartment syndrome develops from lack of tissue perfusion as pressure increases within a fascial compartment, placing muscle and nerve tissue at risk of permanent ischemic damage. Clinically recognizable symptoms, including pain disproportionate to examination, paresthesias, and painful passive motion of fingers and wrist with possible progression to pulselessness, demand prompt treatment with at least volar forearm fasciotomy and low threshold for carpal tunnel release. Although not directly addressing volar plating, Rosenauer and colleagues[9] reported an incidence of 0.25% of compartment syndrome associated with distal radial fractures with a predilection toward patients younger than 35 years and children with a distal radial fracture with an ipsilateral arm fracture. Deep infection after volar plating of distal radial fractures is uncommon. Alter and colleagues[5] found a deep infection rate of 0.03% in reviewing 55 articles on volar plating of distal radial fractures with greater than 12 months' follow-up. Lee and colleagues[10] reported a deep infection rate of 0.10% and a superficial infection rate of 4.25% in 1955 patients with volar plating. It is noteworthy that this infection rate is less than the infection rate associated with unburied Kirschner wires, external fixator pins, or buried Kirschner wires, which have reported infection rates of 33%, 21%, and 7%, respectively.[28] Infection should be prevented by sterile surgical technique, preoperative antibiotic administration, and careful intraoperative hemostasis to prevent bacterial seeding of a hematoma. Deep infection requires formal operative debridement and empiric versus culture-directed antibiotic treatment typically intravenously for several weeks. Later implant removal may be required for complete eradication of the infection.

Operative treatment of displaced distal radial fractures with volar plating has arisen as a popular and effective treatment tool. Potential complications of this treatment should be understood by the treating surgeon with the goal of minimizing adverse outcomes. Although the overall complication rate approaches 15%, less than 5% require reoperation.[5,6] Certain factors involving the patient, the fracture, and/or the surgeon may affect the overall complication risk. Patient factors, including body mass index greater than 35 and diabetes mellitus, may increase complication risk with volar plating,[7] but older patient age does not seem to significantly alter risk.[7,8,10] More severe fractures (such as AO type C fractures, open fractures, and fractures with lunate facet impaction) as well as fractures stabilized with prominent plates may have higher complication rates.[7,25] More complications are also associated with low-volume surgeons.[25,26] Discussing possible complications relating to nerve, tendon, implant, bone/joint, and vessels, surgeons may better inform patients of operative risks and take measures to avoid preventable complications and improve surgical outcomes.

CLINICS CARE POINTS

- Patients may be informed that volar plating carries a 5% risk of a major complication requiring repeat surgery
- Carpal tunnel syndrome is the most common overall complication with surgical release eventually required in 2-3% of patients
- Tendon rupture is possible but rare after volar plating with less than 1-2% for flexor and extensor tendons
- Implants are typically left in place with around 6% requiring removal
- Deep infection is well under 1% of cases

DISCLOSURE

Neither the authors nor their immediate families received any financial payments or other benefits from any commercial entity related to this article.

REFERENCES

1. Karl JW, Olson PR, Rosenwasser MP. The epidemiology of upper extremity fractures in the United States, 2009. J Orthop Trauma 2015;29(8):e242–4.
2. Shauver MJ, Yin H, Banerjee M, et al. Current and future national costs to Medicare for the treatment of distal radius fracture in the elderly. J Hand Surg Am 2011;36(8):1282–7.
3. Ali Fazal M, Denis Mitchell C, Ashwood N. Volar locking plate: Age related outcomes and complications. J Clin Orthop Trauma 2020;11(4):642–5.
4. Huetteman HE, Shauver MJ, Malay S, et al. Variation in the treatment of distal radius fractures in the United States: 2010 to 2015. Plast Reconstr Surg 2019;143(1):159–67.
5. Alter TH, Sandrowski K, Gallant G, et al. Complications of volar plating of distal radius fractures: a systematic review. J Wrist Surg 2019;8(3):255–62.
6. Alter TH, Ilyas AM. Complications associated with volar locking plate fixation of distal radial fractures. JBJS Rev 2018;6(10):e7.
7. DeGeorge BR Jr, Brogan DM, Becker HA, et al. Incidence of complications following volar locking plate fixation of distal radius fractures: an analysis of 647 cases. Plast Reconstr Surg 2020;145(4):969–76.
8. Quadlbauer S, Pezzei C, Jurkowitsch J, et al. Early complications and radiological outcome after distal radius fractures stabilized by volar angular stable locking plate. Arch Orthop Trauma Surg 2018;138(12):1773–82.
9. Rosenauer R, Pezzei C, Quadlbauer S, et al. Complications after operatively treated distal radius fractures. Arch Orthop Trauma Surg 2020;140(5):665–73.
10. Lee JH, Lee JK, Park JS, et al. Complications associated with volar locking plate fixation for distal radius fractures in 1955 cases: A multicentre retrospective study. Int Orthop 2020;44(10):2057–67.
11. Lizaur-Utrilla A, Martinez-Mendez D, Vizcaya-Moreno MF, et al. Volar plate for intra-articular distal radius fracture. A prospective comparative study between elderly and young patients. Orthop Traumatol Surg Res 2020;106(2):319–23.
12. Thorninger T, Madsen ML, Waever D, et al. Complications of volar locking plating of distal radius fractures in 576 patients with 3.2 years follow-up. Injury 2017;48:1104–9.
13. Ojha MM, Agrawal AC, Kar BK, et al. Complications of distal radius fractures. J Orthop Dis Traumatol 2020;3:58–60.
14. Goebel A, Bisla J, Carganillo R, et al. A randomised placebo-controlled Phase III multicentre trial: low-dose intravenous immunoglobulin treatment for long-standing complex regional pain syndrome (LIPS trial). Southampton (UK): NIHR Journals Library; 2017 (Efficacy and Mechanism Evaluation, No. 4.5.) Appendix 3, Research diagnostic criteria (the 'Budapest Criteria') for complex regional pain

syndrome. Available at: https://www.ncbi.nlm.nih.gov/books/NBK464482/.

15. Placzek JD, Boyer MI, Gelberman RH, et al. Nerve decompression for complex regional pain syndrome type II following upper extremity surgery. J Hand Surg Am 2005;30(1):69–74.

16. Fardellas A, Vernet P, Facca S, et al. Flexor tendon complications in distal radius fractures treated with volar rim locking plates. Hand Surg Rehabil 2020;39(6):511–5.

17. Soong M, Earp BE, Bishop G, et al. Volar locking plate implant prominence and flexor tendon rupture. J Bone Joint Surg Am 2011;93:328–35.

18. Yamak K, Karahan HG, Karatan B, et al. Evaluation of flexor pollicis longus tendon rupture after treatment of distal radius fracture with the volar plate. J Wrist Surg 2020;9(3):219–24.

19. Selles CA, Reerds STH, Roukema G, et al. Relationship between plate removal and Soong grading following surgery for fractured distal radius. J Hand Surg Eur Vol 2018;43(2):137–41.

20. Hirasawa R, Itadera E, Okamoto S. Changes in the rate of postoperative flexor tendon rupture in patients with distal radius fractures. J Hand Surg Asian Pac Vol 2020;25(4):481–8.

21. Cook A, Baldwin P, Fowler JR. Incidence of flexor pollicis longus complications following volar locking plate fixation of distal radius fractures. Hand (N Y) 2020;15(5):692–7.

22. Ohno K, Takigawa N, Watanabe C, et al. Effect of downsized screw selection on bone healing and postoperative complications in volar plating of distal radius fractures. Orthopedics 2020;1–7. https://doi.org/10.3928/01477447-20201210-08.

23. Vaiss L, Ichihara S, Hendriks S, et al. The utility of the fluoroscopic skyline view during volar locking plate fixation of distal radius fractures. J Wrist Surg 2014;3(4):245–9.

24. Pidgeon TS, Casey P, Baumgartner RE, et al. Complications of volar locked plating of distal radius fractures: a prospective investigation of modern techniques. Hand (N Y) 2020;15(5):698–706.

25. Li Y, Zhou Y, Zhang X, et al. Incidence of complications and secondary procedure following distal radius fractures treated by volar locking plate (VLP). J Orthop Surg Res 2019;14(1):295.

26. Sirniö K, Flinkkilä T, Vähäkuopus M, et al. Risk factors for complications after volar plate fixation of distal radial fractures. J Hand Surg Eur Vol 2019;44(5):456–61.

27. Dillingham C, Horodyski MB, Struk AM, et al. Rate of improvement following volar plate open reduction and internal fixation of distal radius fractures. Adv Orthop 2011;2011:565642.

28. Mathews AL, Chung KC. Management of complications of distal radius fractures. Hand Clin 2015;31(2):205–15.

Shoulder and Elbow

Acromion and Scapular Spine Fractures Following Reverse Total Shoulder Arthroplasty

Eileen M. Colliton, MD[a], Andrew Jawa, MD[b,c,*],
Jacob M. Kirsch, MD[b,c]

KEYWORDS

- Reverse total shoulder arthroplasty • Complications • Acromion fractures
- Scapular spine fractures • Stress fracture

KEY POINTS

- Although infrequent in overall incidence, postoperative acromion or scapular spine fractures are among the most common complication to occur following reverse shoulder arthroplasty.
- Fracture should be suspected in patients who present with pain postoperatively, and workup should include plain radiographs and computed tomographic scan if indicated.
- Treatment options include nonoperative management in an abduction sling, but open reduction and internal fixation should be considered in patients with symptomatic nonunions after failed nonoperative treatment, or acute fractures with significant displacement and decreased shoulder function.
- Similar clinical outcomes can be achieved following operative and nonoperative treatment.
- Clinical outcomes for patients with acromion or scapular spine fractures are worse than those without fracture but are improved when compared with preoperative function.

INTRODUCTION

Reverse total shoulder arthroplasty (RSA) was originally indicated for severe rotator cuff tear arthropathy (CTA). Utilization of RSA has continued to expand as indications have broadened to include diagnoses, such as glenohumeral arthritis, proximal humerus fracture, failed anatomic total shoulder arthroplasty, and fracture sequelae.[1] With the growing number of RSAs being performed, various complications are more frequently encountered; however, the rates of complication and reoperation are low with modern implant designs and techniques.[2,3] The most common complications include instability, fracture, hematoma, heterotopic ossification, deltoid injury, complex regional pain syndrome, and postoperative acromial or scapular spine fractures. Acromion and scapular spine fractures are uncommon in overall incidence but can significantly impact clinical outcomes. The function of the shoulder after RSA is largely dependent on a functional deltoid; therefore, a fracture of the acromion or scapular spine has the potential to significantly impact the overall stability and function of the shoulder.[4] Various studies have investigated the incidence, pathophysiology, risk factors, treatment options, and outcomes associated with acromion and scapular spine fractures following RSA. In this article, the authors review the current available literature.

[a] Department of Orthopaedic Surgery, Tufts Medical Center, 800 Washington Street, Boston, MA 02111, USA; [b] Department of Orthopaedic Surgery, New England Baptist Hospital, 125 Parker Hill Avenue, Boston, MA 02120, USA; [c] Boston Sports and Shoulder Center, 840 Winter Street, Waltham, MA 02451, USA
* Corresponding author.
E-mail address: andrewjawa@gmail.com

Orthop Clin N Am 52 (2021) 257–268
https://doi.org/10.1016/j.ocl.2021.03.006

INCIDENCE

Acromion and scapular spine fractures have a variable incidence in the literature, from 0.8% to 11.2%,[2,5–23] with acromion fractures being more common than scapular spine fractures.[2,19,23] Mahendraraj and colleagues[23] conducted a multicenter retrospective review of more than 6000 RSAs and found a 3.0% incidence of acromial fracture and a 0.9% incidence of scapular spine fracture, totaling a 3.9% incidence of stress fracture overall. A recent systematic review of 32 studies with more than 3800 RSAs identified 159 fractures of the acromion or scapular spine, resulting in an incidence of 4.14%.[24] A second recent systematic review of 90 studies found an overall incidence of 2.8% for acromial or scapular spine fractures,[25] similar to the 2.6% incidence identified in the systematic review by Shah and colleagues[2] of more than 14,000 RSAs with modern prosthesis design.

The variation in reported incidence may be due to various factors, including underlying diagnosis, patient factors, implant geometry/design, and inconsistent diagnosis. Zmistowski and colleagues[26] identified many patients with pain and point tenderness over the acromion suspicious for a stress fracture with negative radiographs, which was termed a "stress reaction." In their review of approximately 1000 cases, they found a 10.5% incidence of either radiographically diagnosed acromial fracture or symptoms suspicious for acromial injury. In total, 4.2% of patients were identified to have a definitive stress fracture on radiographs, whereas 6.4% were identified as a stress reaction, with no acute findings on radiographs. In the retrospective study by Otto and colleagues,[27] 32% of patients presenting with pain had negative radiographs but were then identified as having a periscapular fracture later in their clinical course, with approximately 79% of fractures being diagnosed by plain radiograph. The difficulty in diagnosing acromion and scapular spine fractures after RSA suggests that reported incidence in the literature may underrepresent the true rate of occurrence.

DIAGNOSIS

A high degree of clinical suspicion is necessary to accurately diagnose acromion and scapular spine fractures. Surgeons should have a low threshold to obtain additional imaging to aid in the diagnosis, as timely intervention is important. Patients with acromion or scapular spine fractures following RSA often present with increased pain along the acromion with tenderness to palpation and decreased shoulder function.[28] If these symptoms are seen, a plain radiograph should be obtained to assess for a fracture.[28] Often these fractures are difficult to see on plain radiograph with metallic implants obstructing clear view of the acromion, or will not be seen on initial presentation, but will be identified on later radiograph with fracture displacement.[19,27] Increasing acromial tilt and decreasing acromion-to-tuberosity distance on follow-up radiographs in the postoperative period may clue a clinician to a possible fracture[27] (Fig. 1). If a clinician has continued suspicion despite a negative radiograph, a computed tomographic (CT) scan should be obtained for a complete assessment.[28] In the retrospective review by Marigi and colleagues,[19] radiographs identified 61% of fractures, and CT identified the remaining 39% of fractures. It is important to recognize that acromion and scapular spine fractures can occur almost any time in the postoperative period,[14] with reported mean time to diagnosis of 3.3 to 38 months, with reported range of time to diagnosis of 1 to 66 months.[11–13,17–19,21,24,27,29] Given this broad timeframe, the diagnosis of acromion or scapular spine fracture should always be on the differential when a patient presents with pain following RSA.

CLASSIFICATION

There are 2 main classification systems that have been designed for acromion and scapular spine fractures following RSA: the Levy[10] classification system and the Crosby[6] classification system.

Levy Classification
Levy and colleagues[10] completed a retrospective review and created a classification system for acromial fractures based on the origin of the deltoid (Fig. 2). Type I includes fracture of the anterior and middle origin of the deltoid; type II includes fracture of the entire middle origin of the deltoid, and type III includes fracture of the middle and posterior origin of the deltoid.[10] Most studies identify Levy type I and II fractures to occur with relatively equal frequency, and both to be more common than Levy type III fractures.[12,13,16,19,26]

Crosby Classification
Crosby and colleagues[6] completed a retrospective review of 400 RSA patients and developed a classification system for acromion and scapula

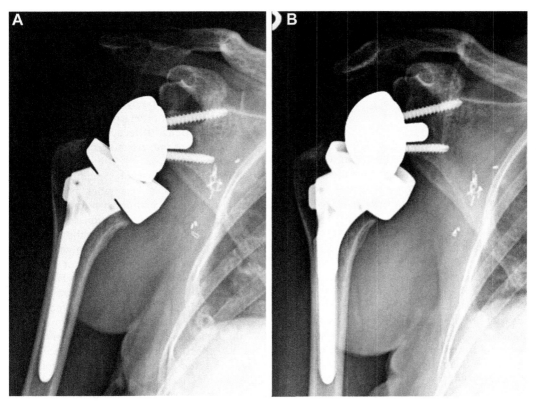

Fig. 1. The interval change in anteroposterior (AP) radiographs following RSA suggestive of postoperative acromial or scapular spine fracture. (*A*) AP view of the right shoulder postoperatively following RSA. (*B*) AP view of the right shoulder 3 months postoperatively in the same patient. There is increased acromial tilt and decreased acromion-to-tuberosity distance, suggesting a possible fracture.

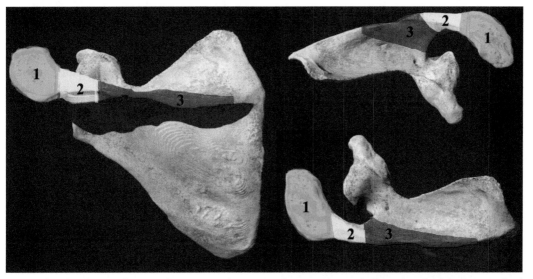

Fig. 2. The classification for scapular spine and acromion fractures (types 1–3) as described by Levy and colleagues,[10] including a posterior view (*left*), superior view (*upper right*), and oblique posterior superior view (*lower right*). (*Modified from* "Left Scapula" from the anthropology department's collections at University of North Carolina at Greensboro, modeled with the permission of Dr Robert Anemone, created by Cory Henderson; Licensed under Creative Commons Attribution. https://skfb.ly/MusD To view a copy of this license, visit http://creativecommons.org/licenses/by/4.0/.)

fractures. Their fracture classification consisted of type I iatrogenic anterior acromial avulsion fractures, type II anterior acromial fractures posterior to the acromioclavicular (AC) joint, and type III scapular spine or posterior acromial fractures.[6] Most studies identify Crosby type II and III fractures at relatively equal frequency.[12,19]

CAUSE

Various factors have been associated with acromial and scapular spine stress fractures. Among the most common are patient factors (gender/bone quality), underlying diagnosis, implant design/geometry, altered shoulder biomechanics, and load transfer with RSA and technical surgical factors.

Biomechanics of Reverse Shoulder Arthroplasty

RSA design allows the deltoid to compensate for a deficient rotator cuff by moving the center of rotation (COR) distal and medial, tensioning the deltoid, and providing an effective lever arm for the deltoid to facilitate shoulder range of motion.[30] As the deltoid assumes a larger role for shoulder flexion and abduction, the acromion experiences increased stress.[31] In addition, distalization of the COR lengthens the arm and tensions the deltoid, whereas medialization of the COR results in a more vertical line of pull for the deltoid.[17] This combination results in an increased bending force on the acromion following RSA,[17,19] which can increase the risk of fracture. In support of this mechanism, acromial fracture has been found to be associated with deltoid lengthening in retrospective studies.[17]

Shah and colleagues[32] conducted a cadaveric study to determine the relationship between deltoid lengthening and acromion and scapular strain. They found that deltoid lengthening is linearly correlated with acromial strain, and the observed strain values were significant enough to cause microscopic damage, which may lead to fatigue fractures over time.[32] In addition, the orientation of the acromion was found to play a role in strain patterns, with a more posterior orientation resulting in the scapular spine experiencing more strain from deltoid lengthening, and more anterior orientation resulting in the acromion experiencing more strain from deltoid lengthening.[32]

Preoperative Shoulder Pathologic Condition

Shoulder pathologic condition commonly found in patients undergoing RSA is also thought to play a role in the development of acromial and scapular spine fractures. In the retrospective review by Routman and colleagues,[16] patients with acromion or scapular spine fractures postoperatively were significantly more likely to have rheumatoid arthritis and rotator cuff arthropathy. Rotator cuff arthropathy, which is a common indication for RSA, often produces osteoporotic acromions in patients because of disuse, resulting in acromions that are more prone to fracture with increased stress.[31,33,34] In addition, some have hypothesized that rotator cuff injury results in changes in scapular kinematics, increasing the activity of muscles that insert or originate from the scapular spine or acromion to help with arm elevation, further increasing the stress that the scapula experiences with arm motion.[11,35] What remains of the intact rotator cuff may play a role in the location of acromial erosion, with an intact subscapularis tendon resulting in more posterior acromion erosion, affecting the base of the acromion or scapular spine.[11] When both the subscapularis and the infraspinatus are intact, shoulders have been shown to have increased adduction capabilities following RSA, thereby increasing the joint reaction force and the force required of the deltoid for shoulder range of motion.[16]

Acromion weakening from previous surgery (such as acromioplasty) or from wear (such as from the humeral head in CTA) can also place the acromion at risk for fracture[27]; however, retrospective reviews by Walch and colleagues[15] and Werner and colleagues[36] have found no difference in postoperative RSA outcomes when comparing patients with and without preoperative acromial stress fractures or alternative pathologic condition. These investigative findings may be because tensioning during surgery already accounts for the acromial pathologic condition present preoperatively.[36]

In the retrospective review by Crosby and colleagues,[6] type II fractures, or anterior acromial fractures posterior to the AC joint, were thought to be related to significant AC joint arthrosis and stiffness resulting in increased stress through the acromion with shoulder range of motion postoperatively. A retrospective review by Dubrow and colleagues,[18] however, did not find an association between AC joint arthritis and postoperative acromial stress fracture.

Baseplate Fixation

A potential mechanism for periprosthetic scapular spine fracture includes stress risers from baseplate screws[19] (Fig. 3). In the retrospective review by Crosby and colleagues,[6] type III

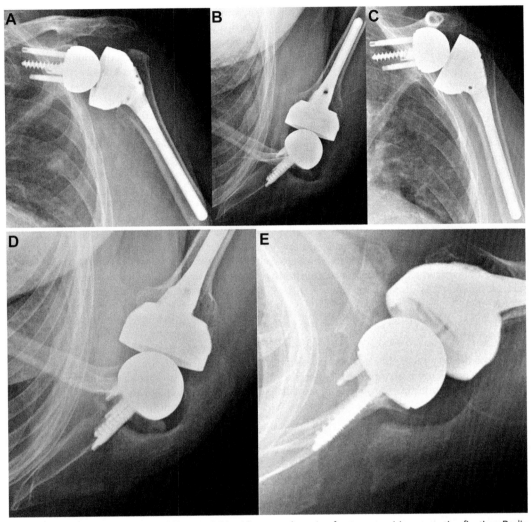

Fig. 3. Postoperative radiographs following RSA with a scapular spine fracture requiring operative fixation. Radiographs are from a female patient with a history of rheumatoid arthritis and rotator cuff arthropathy. (*A, B*) The AP and axillary lateral postoperative shoulder radiographs following RSA. (*C, D*) The AP and axillary lateral radiographs 3 months postoperatively, demonstrating a Levy III/scapular spine fracture adjacent to glenoid baseplate screw fixation. (*E*) A repeat axillary lateral 7 months postoperatively demonstrating interval widening of the fracture site and coracoid displacement.

fractures, or scapular spine or posterior acromial fractures, were thought to be related to trauma in combination with superior glenoid screw fixation, causing a stress riser. Levy and Blum[28] also proposed that fractures at the base of the acromion may be related to baseplate screw fixation in the posterior-superior quadrant, resulting in a stress riser at the acromial base. Ascione and colleagues[5] conducted a retrospective review of 485 RSA cases and found that 57% of scapular spine fractures occurred at the tip of the superior glenoid fixation screw. Otto and colleagues[27] also conducted a retrospective study and found that 14 of 16 scapular spine fractures occurred in association with glenoid screw placement, 11 of which were posterior-superior. The retrospective review by Routman and colleagues[16] reported the number of baseplate screws was significantly associated with fracture, with more fixation (4.1 screws) being seen in the fracture group when compared with the nonfracture group (3.8 screws). A retrospective review by Kennon and colleagues[9] found that avoiding use of the superior baseplate screw decreased the occurrence of fracture in the scapular spine from 4.4% to 0%. It is important to ensure the glenoid baseplate has secure fixation to prevent glenoid component loosening; however, these studies also demonstrate the importance of being mindful of screw location and length when obtaining peripheral fixation.

Mechanical Falls

Traumatic injuries have also been found to be associated with acromion and scapular spine fractures following RSA. Hattrup[8] conducted a retrospective review and found that fall was the most common cause of fracture. The retrospective review by Nyffeler and colleagues[21] also found that most cases of acromion or scapular spine fracture following RSA were secondary to falls. They hypothesized that medialization and distalization of the humerus make the acromion more prominent and thus more susceptible to fracture with falls.[21] In the multicenter retrospective study by Mahendraraj and colleagues,[23] scapular spine fractures were found to be associated with trauma more often than acromion stress fractures (33% vs 18%, respectively).

RISK FACTORS

Because acromion and scapular spine fractures after RSA can have potential detrimental effects to shoulder stability and function, multiple studies have attempted to determine risk factors associated with this postoperative complication. Many risk factors have been identified in the literature, including a history of previous surgery, such as acromioplasty,[17,19] female gender,[16,19,20,23,26] low bone mineral density,[13,17,19,20,22,23,26,27] arm or deltoid lengthening,[13,17] history of inflammatory arthritis,[2,16,20,23,25] thinning acromion,[13,37] large rotator cuff tears or rotator cuff arthropathy,[16,20,23,25] posterosuperior position of the superior glenoid baseplate screw,[11,16] older age,[23] chronic dislocation,[23] and malunion or nonunion.[20]

Cho and colleagues[17] conducted a retrospective case-control study of almost 800 patients who underwent RSA and found acromial fractures to be associated with a history of previous surgery, a low bone mineral density, and deltoid lengthening. The retrospective review of more than 1000 shoulders by Werthel and colleagues[13] similarly found osteoporosis, thinner acromion, and arm lengthening to be risk factors for acromial fracture following RSA. Marigi and colleagues[19] also conducted a retrospective review of more than 2000 RSAs and used multivariate regression analysis to determine the risk of scapular fractures postoperatively. No significant risk factors were identified; however, there was a trend toward increased risk of fracture in women with osteopenia and a history of

acromioplasty.[19] They found no correlation with age, body mass index, history of rotator cuff repair, or surgical indication.[19] Moverman and colleagues[20] conducted a multicenter retrospective study of approximately 1500 patients undergoing primary or revision RSA, and through multivariable logistic regression identified female sex, decreased bone stock, rheumatoid arthritis, rotator cuff arthropathy and malunion or nonunion as risk factors for acromial fracture postoperatively. These findings were similar to the risk factors identified in the retrospective review of more than 4000 shoulders by Routman and colleagues,[16] which found significantly higher rates of fracture in women, patients with rheumatoid arthritis, patients with rotator cuff arthropathy, and patients with more baseplate screws. Mahendraraj and colleagues[23] conducted a multicenter retrospective study of more than 6000 RSAs and through multivariable regression analysis identified chronic dislocation, large rotator cuff tear, rotator cuff arthropathy, osteoporosis, female sex, inflammatory arthritis, and older age as independent risk factors for acromial stress fracture. When looking at scapular spine fractures, the same study identified osteoporosis, female sex, inflammatory arthritis, and rotator cuff arthropathy as independent risk factors.[23] RSA for osteoarthritis may actually have fewer stress fracture than RSA for other surgical indications.

Contrary to the above studies, Otto and colleagues[27] found no significant relationship between acromial bone thickness and risk of osteoporotic fracture, and Dubrow and colleagues[18] found no significant relationship between distalization and acromial stress fracture. In addition, Zmistowski and colleagues[26] and Schenk and colleagues[22] found in their individual retrospective reviews of approximately 1000 cases that decreased deltoid lengthening, instead of increased lengthening, was actually a risk factor for acromial fracture after RSA. They reported that decreased deltoid lengthening possibly created a mechanical disadvantage, resulting in increased forces necessary for arm range of motion, thereby putting more stress on the acromion.[26]

ASSOCIATION WITH IMPLANT DESIGN

As stated previously, the RSA design works by moving the shoulder COR distal and medial, tensioning the deltoid and providing an effective lever arm for the deltoid to facilitate shoulder function.[30] More modern RSA implants have trended toward moving the COR more lateral when compared with the tradition Grammont-style prosthesis to decrease the incidence of scapular notching, improve range of motion, and improve soft tissue tensioning and stability.[30,38] Various studies have looked at the impact different RSA implant designs have on acromion and scapular spine fractures following RSA.

Protective Effect of Humeral Lateralization

Some studies have shown that a lateralized humeral component is associated with a decreased risk for acromial or scapular spine fractures following RSA. Cho and colleagues[17] conducted a retrospective review of more than 700 cases and found a significant association between implant design and acromial fractures after RSA, with medialized glenoid and medialized humerus designs resulting in an 8.4% incidence of acromion fractures, and medialized glenoid and lateralized humerus resulting in a 2.8% incidence. These findings suggest that a more modern lateralized humerus in combination with a medial glenoid may have a protective effect against acromial fractures. Routman and colleagues[16] conducted a retrospective review of more than 4000 RSAs with only medialized glenoid and lateralized humeral implants and found a 1.77% incidence of scapular and acromial fractures postoperatively and that combined humeral tray and liner offset was larger in the nonfracture group when compared with the fracture group; however, results did not reach statistical significance on multivariate analysis. The retrospective reviews by Schenk and colleagues[22] and Werthel and colleagues[13] also found that increased COR medialization was a risk factor for postoperative acromial fracture, suggesting lateralization of the humerus has a protective effect by increasing the mechanical advantage of the deltoid. King and colleagues[25] investigated the role of prosthetic design on risk of acromial or scapular spine fracture using a meta-analysis and similarly found that a medialized glenoid component with a lateralized humeral component had the lowest risk of fracture (1.5%). They thought these findings were likely due to a lateralized humeral component's association with improved efficiency of the deltoid with a larger abduction moment arm.[25] A significantly higher rate of fractures was found for lateralized glenoid and medialized humerus designs (3.8%).[25] These results are similar to the findings described by Shah and colleagues,[2] who found the highest incidence of fracture with lateralized glenoid and medialized humerus designs, and the lowest risk of

fracture with medialized glenoid and lateralized humerus designs. Lateralizing the glenoid component decreases the abduction moment arm of the deltoid and thereby increased the deltoid force necessary with arm elevation, which may increase stress on the scapula and thus result in an increased risk of fracture.[25]

Combined Distalization and Lateralization as a Risk Factor

On the other hand, other studies have suggested that a lateralized and distalized humeral onlay prosthesis may be associated with an increased risk for acromial or scapular spine fracture following RSA. Neyton and colleagues[12] found a 1.3% rate of scapular fracture with Grammont-style prosthesis. This incidence is markedly lower than the 4.3%[5] and 5.3%[39] incidence reported by other studies using lateralized and distalized onlay prosthesis, suggesting that an onlay stem may be associated with the higher incidence of postoperative scapular spine or acromial fractures following RSA. Haidamous and colleagues[40] conducted a retrospective review to look at the effects of distalization and lateralization on scapular spine fractures and found a 2.5 times higher risk of scapular spine fractures with onlay stems, which were found to increase distalization by 10 mm and double offset when compared with inlay stems. In addition, distalization was found to increase the risk of scapular spine fracture postoperatively.[40] A cadaveric study by Shah and colleagues[32] investigated the relationship between deltoid lengthening and acromion strain with various implant designs. They found that both humeral and glenoid lateralization significantly lengthened the deltoid through distalization, and acromion strain increased with increasing lateralization of the humerus.[32] In addition, with each humeral condition, glenosphere lateralization further increased acromion strain.[32] Wong and colleagues[41] similarly used a 3-dimensional model to evaluate acromial stresses with various RSA implant positions and found acromial stress increased by 17% with glenosphere lateralization, while medialization of the glenosphere allows for recruitment of anterior and posterior deltoid fibers, resulting in a larger distribution of stress.

Lack of Association Between Fracture and Implant Design

In contrast to the studies mentioned above, some reviews found no association between implant design and risk of acromion or scapular spine fracture following RSA. Marigi and colleagues[19] conducted a multivariate regression analysis of more than 2000 RSAs and found no significant correlation between scapular spine or acromion fractures with implant design or size. Shah and colleagues[2] and Zmistowski and colleagues[26] similarly found no significant difference in the rate of fracture when comparing different combinations of implant designs.

TREATMENT

Acromion or scapular spine fractures following RSA have the potential to cause significant shoulder pain and dysfunction.[7,17] Pull of the deltoid through the fracture can result in inferior tilt of the acromion, which can compromise function and shoulder stability.[28] Acromion or scapular spine fractures with inferior displacement may reduce the deltoid resting tension and thereby decrease shoulder abduction and forward elevation.[31] In addition, instability can result because of loss of the soft tissue compressive force from the deltoid.[28] Described treatment options for acromial and scapular spine fractures following RSA include no intervention, sling immobilization, and open reduction internal fixation.

No Intervention

Asymptomatic, incidental acromion fractures identified on routine postoperative radiographs are generally managed without any specific intervention. In a retrospective review by Boileau and colleagues,[34] 45 patients were evaluated following Grammont-style RSA, and at 3 months' follow-up, 2 patients were found to have asymptomatic acromial fractures identified incidentally on postoperative radiographs. No significant negative effects on patient outcomes or range of motion were identified. For these asymptomatic patients, treatment is likely not needed; however, close observation is warranted.[31]

Sling Immobilization

Conservative management has been recommended for symptomatic acromial fractures, as these can usually be successfully managed with nonoperative treatment.[8,15,42,43] Conservative treatment generally consists of 6 weeks of immobilization in an abduction sling.[12,14–16,19,24] Increased shoulder abduction is used to take some of the tension out of the deltoid to theoretically reduce the downward pull on the acromion. Symptomatic nonunion necessitating surgical fixation can occur.[12,24] Neyton and colleagues[12] conducted a retrospective review of

approximately 1000 RSAs and identified 10 acromial base and 9 scapular spine fractures postoperatively. Symptomatic patients were treated with immobilization, resulting in 40% of acromial fractures healing, and 33% of scapular spine fractures healing, correlating to a nonunion rate of 66%.[12] Two scapular spine fractures subsequently had surgical treatment.[12] Patterson and colleagues[24] conducted a systematic review to evaluate the outcomes of acromial spine fractures following RSA. Reported union rates varied from 50% to 60% with nonoperative management, and they found that pain and dysfunction of the shoulder improved for fractures that achieved union with nonoperative management.[24]

Operative Treatment

Open reduction and internal fixation can be considered for scapular spine fractures, as these are typically displaced and painful.[8,15,42,43] In addition, it is reasonable to consider fixation for fractures involving most of the deltoid insertion (ie, scapular spine or base of the acromion) because of the possible negative impact on function and implant stability without fixation[11] (Figs. 3–5). Preoperative bone thinning and osteoporosis are common in this population; thus, the bone stock available for internal fixation is often poor, making fixation difficult.[8,15] Fixation will also need to withstand significant load from contraction of the deltoid, adding further difficulty to obtaining a stable construct.[8,15] In addition, although fixation has been suggested for displaced fractures impacting a significant portion of the deltoid, improved outcomes have not been shown with operative fixation.[2,44] Wahlquist and colleagues[45] reported on a series of acromion base fractures where the entire origin of the deltoid was displaced. Half were managed nonoperatively in a sling, and half were managed operatively with fixation.[45] Both operative and nonoperative treatment had inconsistent results with no predictable functional outcomes; however, both strategies for treatment effectively decreased pain and increased range of motion as the fracture healed.[45]

In cases of shoulder instability owing to loss of soft tissue and deltoid tension secondary to base of acromion or scapular spine fracture, revision RSA with a larger glenosphere and humeral augmentation can be considered to increase soft tissue tensioning and provide shoulder stability if the acromial fracture is not thought to be amenable to internal fixation.[28]

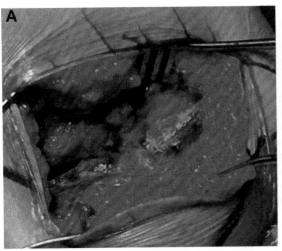
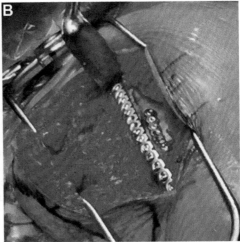

Fig. 4. Intraoperative photographs demonstrating open reduction and internal fixation of an unstable Levy III/scapular spine fracture. (A) An intraoperative photograph showing the fracture site. (B) An intraoperative photograph showing the reduced fracture after internal fixation.

Treatment by Fracture Classification

The classification system designed by Crosby and colleagues[6] attempted to outline treatment recommendations for acromion and scapular fractures based on review of 400 patients. Crosby type I fractures were thought to be benign, and all were managed successfully nonoperatively.[6] Nonoperative treatment of Crosby type II fractures can be considered in patients who are low demand or poor surgical candidates with the understanding that future displacement is possible with persistent pain.[6] AC joint resection was considered a treatment option for stable Crosby type II fractures to allow dissipation of acromial stresses and fracture healing,[6] and for unstable Crosby type II fractures, surgical fixation was considered with possible AC joint resection.[6] Surgical treatment was also considered for all unstable Crosby type III fractures.[6] Using these principles, in their review of 400 patients, all surgically treated fractures united with resolution of pain.[6]

The authors' current practice is to manage Levy I and II fractures nonoperatively and only consider operative intervention if the patient experiences significant pain, shoulder dysfunction,

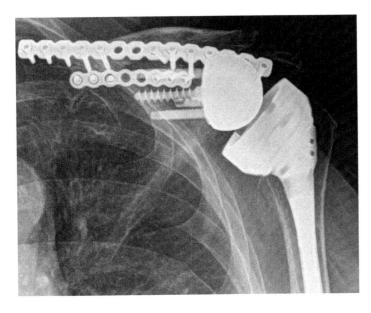

Fig. 5. Postoperative AP radiograph of the shoulder following open reduction and internal fixation of an unstable Levy III/scapular spine fracture.

or instability. The authors recommend open reduction and internal fixation for acute Levy III fractures.

OUTCOMES

Multiple studies have evaluated clinical outcomes for patients with and without acromion or scapular spine fractures following RSA. Most studies have found that patients with acromion or scapular spine fractures had improved outcomes when compared with their preoperative state; however, outcomes are generally worse when compared with those patients without fracture postoperatively.[5,8,11,12,14–17]

In the retrospective review by Cho and colleagues,[17] 69% of patients with acromial fractures postoperatively had pain and decreased range of motion, whereas 27% had only pain, and 3% had no symptoms. Dubrow and colleagues[18] conducted a retrospective review and found that patients with acromial stress fractures had significantly decreased forward elevation when compared with those without fracture (116° vs 143°) but reported similar clinical outcome scores between the 2 groups. In the retrospective studies by Ascione and colleagues,[5] Teusink and colleagues,[14] Lópiz and colleagues,[11] and Hattrup,[8] significant differences in clinical outcome scores, abduction, and forward flexion were found when comparing patients with and without acromion or scapular spine fractures. Despite the decreased relative postoperative outcomes, patients with stress fractures demonstrated improvement when compared with their preoperative function. Similarly, Routman and colleagues[16] found improved clinical outcomes, abduction, internal rotation, and forward elevation in patients without acromial or scapular stress fractures. Patterson and colleagues[24] reported inferior clinical results after acromial spine fracture when compared with outcomes before fracture and outcomes for patients without fracture.[24] Forward flexion, abduction, and clinical outcome scores, such as Constant score and ASES, were the most severely affected, and patients whose fractures healed had improved function when compared with those who went on to nonunion. Levy type I or III fractures have been shown to have worst outcomes,[10,24] and scapular spine fractures have been shown to have worse clinical outcomes and forward elevation when compared with patients with acromial fracture.[15] In contrast, a retrospective study by Werthel and colleagues[13] of more than 1000 RSAs found patients with and without acromial fracture to have comparable results in terms of postoperative pain relief, range of motion, and clinical outcomes; however, patients with fracture reported less satisfaction.

SUMMARY

Acromion and scapular spine fractures are a rare but potentially debilitating complication following RSA. Given the importance of the deltoid for RSA mechanics, fracture of the acromion or scapular spine can significantly impact shoulder function and stability. Fracture should be suspected in any patient who presents with localized pain and decreased shoulder function after RSA, especially if they are female and have a history of osteoporosis, rotator cuff arthropathy, or inflammatory arthritis, regardless of whether there is a history of trauma. Workup should include plain radiographs, and a CT scan if radiographs are negative but clinical presentation is still concerning. For patients with asymptomatic fractures, treatment is likely not indicated; however, close clinical observation is necessary. Symptomatic patients should be managed with an abduction sling for approximately 6 weeks. Operative treatment with open reduction and internal fixation should be considered for patients with symptomatic nonunions after nonoperative management, and for acute traumatic fractures involving a large portion of the deltoid origin with significant displacement. When considering operative management, the patient's bone stock and the amount of stress the fixation construct will experience postoperatively should be factored into the shared decision-making process. Patients should be counseled that although their clinical outcomes and range of motion will be improved when compared with their preoperative status, their outcomes will likely not be as good as those without fracture.

CLINICS CARE POINTS

- Acromion and scapular spine fractures should be considered in the differential diagnosis for patients presenting with shoulder pain and dysfunction following RSA.
- Work-up should include plain radiographs of the shoulders. If the radiographs are negative but there is a high degree of clinical suspicion, a CT scan should be obtained for better evaluation.

- Treatment is often non-operative with sling immobilization; however, open reduction and internal fixation should be considered in patients with acute fractures with significant displacement, and in patients with symptomatic non-union after non-operative management.

DISCLOSURES

No commercial or financial conflicts of interest. No funding sources. Andrew Jawa is a paid speaker and consultant for DJO Global, a paid consultant for Ignite Orthopedics, receives royalties from Depuy Synthesis, and has equity in Boston Outpatient Surgical Suites. Jacob Kirsch, his immediate family, and any research foundation with which he is affiliated did not receive any financial payments or other benefits from any commercial entity related to the subject of this article.

REFERENCES

1. Kurowicki J, Triplet JJ, Momoh E, et al. Reverse shoulder prosthesis in the treatment of locked anterior shoulders: a comparison with classic reverse shoulder indications. J Shoulder Elbow Surg 2016;25:1954–60.
2. Shah SS, Roche AM, Sullivan SW, et al. The modern reverse shoulder arthroplasty and an updated systematic review for each complication: part II. JSES Int 2020;5(1):121–37. https://doi.org/10.1016/j.jseint.2020.07.018.
3. Kang JR, Dubiel MJ, Cofield RH, et al. Primary reverse shoulder arthroplasty using contemporary implants is associated with very low reoperation rates. J Shoulder Elbow Surg 2019;28:S175–80.
4. Ekelund A, Seebauer L. Acromial and scapular spine fractures after reverse shoulder arthroplasty. Obere Extremitat 2017;12:32–7.
5. Ascione F, Kilian CM, Laughlin MS, et al. Increased scapular spine fractures after reverse shoulder arthroplasty with a humeral onlay short stem: an analysis of 485 consecutive cases. J Shoulder Elbow Surg 2018;27:2183–90.
6. Crosby LA, Hamilton A, Twiss T. Scapula fractures after reverse total shoulder arthroplasty: classification and treatment. Clin Orthop Relat Res 2011;469(9):2544–9.
7. Hamid N, Connor PM, Fleischli JF, et al. Acromial fracture after reverse shoulder arthroplasty. Am J Orthop 2011;40(7):E125–9.
8. Hattrup SJ. The influence of postoperative acromial and scapular spine fractures on the results of reverse shoulder arthroplasty. Orthopedics 2010;12:33.
9. Kennon JC, Lu C, McGee-Lawrence ME, et al. Scapula fracture incidence in reverse total shoulder arthroplasty using screws above or below metaglene central cage: clinical and biomechanical outcomes. J Shoulder Elbow Surg 2017;26(6):1023–30.
10. Levy JC, Anderson C, Samson A. Classification of postoperative acromial fractures following reverse shoulder arthroplasty. J Bone Joint Surg Am 2013;95(15):e104.
11. Lópiz Y, Rodríguez-González A, García-Fernández C, et al. Scapula insufficiency fractures after reverse total shoulder arthroplasty in rotator cuff arthropathy: what is their functional impact? Rev Esp Cir Ortop Traumatol 2015;59(5):318–25.
12. Neyton L, Erickson J, Ascione F, et al. Grammont Award 2018: scapular fractures in reverse shoulder arthroplasty (Grammont style): prevalence, functional, and radiographic results with minimum 5-year follow-up. J Shoulder Elbow Surg 2019;28(2):260–7.
13. Werthel JD, Schoch BS, Van Veen SC, et al. Acromial fractures in reverse shoulder arthroplasty: a clinical and radiographic analysis. J Shoulder Elbow Arthroplasty 2018;2:1–9.
14. Teusink MJ, Otto RJ, Cottrell BJ, et al. What is the effect of postoperative scapular fracture on outcomes of reverse shoulder arthroplasty? J Shoulder Elbow Surg 2014;23(6):782–90.
15. Walch G, Mottier F, Wall B, et al. Acromial insufficiency in reverse shoulder arthroplasties. J Shoulder Elbow Surg 2009;18(3):495–502.
16. Routman HD, Simovitch RW, Wright TW, et al. Acromial and scapular fractures after reverse total shoulder arthroplasty with a medialized glenoid and lateralized humeral implant: an analysis of outcomes and risk factors. J Bone Joint Surg Am 2020;102:1724–33.
17. Cho CH, Rhee TG, Yoo JC, et al. Incidence and risk factors of acromial fracture following reverse total shoulder arthroplasty. J Shoulder Elbow Surg 2020;1–8.
18. Dubrow S, Streit JJ, Muh S, et al. Acromion stress fractures: correlation with acromioclavicular osteoarthritis and acromiohumeral distance. Orthopedics 2014;37(12):e1074–9.
19. Marigi E, Bartels D, Tangtiphaiboontana J, et al. Acromial and spine fracture after reverse arthroplasty: prevalence and risk factors. Semin Arthoplasty 2020;30:237–41.
20. Moverman MA, Menendez ME, Mahendraraj KA, et al. Patient risk factors for acromial stress fractures after reverse shoulder arthroplasty: a multicenter study. J Shoulder Elbow Surg 2020. https://doi.org/10.1016/j.jse.2020.09.012.
21. Nyffeler RW, Altioklar B, Bissig P. Causes of acromion and scapular spine fractures following reverse shoulder arthroplasty: a retrospective analysis and literature review. Int Orthop 2020;44:2673–81.

22. Schenk P, Aichmair A, Beeler S, et al. Acromial fractures following reverse total shoulder arthroplasty: a cohort controlled analysis. Orthopedics 2020; 43(1):15–22.

23. Mahendraraj KA, Abboud J, Armstrong A, et al. Predictors of acromial and scapular stress fracture after reverse shoulder arthroplasty: a muticenter study from the ASES acromial stress fracture research group. J Shoulder Elbow Surg 2021.

24. Patterson DC, Chi D, Parsons BO, et al. Acromial spine fracture after reverse total shoulder arthroplasty: a systematic review. J Shoulder Elbow Surg 2019;28:972.

25. King JJ, Dalton SS, Gulotta LV, et al. How common are acromial and scapular spine fractures after reverse shoulder arthroplasty? A systematic review. Bone Joint J 2019;101-B:627–34.

26. Zmistowski B, Gutman M, Horvath Y, et al. Acromial stress fracture following reverse total shoulder arthroplasty: incidence and predictors. J Shoulder Elbow Surg 2020;29:799–806.

27. Otto RJ, Virani NA, Levy JC, et al. Scapular fractures after reserve shoulder arthroplasty: evaluation of risk factors and the reliability of a proposed classification. J Shoulder Elbow Surg 2013;22:1514–21.

28. Levy JC, Blum S. Postoperative acromion base fracture resulting in subsequent instability of reverse shoulder replacement. J Shoulder Elbow Surg 2012;21:e14–8.

29. Werner CML, Steinmann PA, Gilbart M, et al. Treatment of painful pseudoparesis due to irreparable rotator cuff dysfunction with the Delta III reverse-ball-and-socket total shoulder prosthesis. J Bone Joint Surg Am 2005;87A(7):1476–86.

30. Berliner JL, Regalado-Magdos A, Ma CB, et al. Biomechanics of reverse total shoulder arthroplasty. J Shoulder Elbow Surg 2015;24:150–60.

31. Burkholz KJ, Roberts CC, Hattrup SJ. Scapular spine stress fracture as a complication of reverse shoulder arthroplasty. Radiol Case Rep 2007;2(2):78–82.

32. Shah SS, Gentile J, Chen X, et al. Influence of implant design and parasagittal acromial morphology on acromial and scapular spine strain after reverse total shoulder arthroplasty: a cadaveric and computer-based biomechanical analysis. J Shoulder Elbow Surg 2020;29:2395–405.

33. Barco R, Savvidou OD, Sperling JW, et al. Complications in reverse shoulder arthroplasty. Effort Open Rev 2016;1:72–80.

34. Boileau P, Watkinson D, Hatzidakis AM, et al. Neer Award 2005: the Grammont reverse shoulder prosthesis: results in cuff tear arthritis, fracture sequelae, and revision arthroplasty. J Shoulder Elbow Surg 2006;15:527–40.

35. Garciá-Coiradas J, Lópiz Y, Marco F. Fracturas de estrés de la espina de la escápula asociadas a lesion del man- guito rotador: a proposito de 3 casos y revision de la literatura. Rev Esp Cir Ortop Traumatol 2014;58:314–8.

36. Werner BC, Gulotta LV, Dines JS, et al. Acromion comprovise does not significantly affect clinical outcomes after reverse shoulder arthroplasty: a matched case-control study. HSS J 2019;15: 147–52.

37. Yeazell ST, Malige A, Visser T, et al. The role of acromial morphometry in the development of acromial stress fracture following reverse total shoulder arthroplasty. Shoulder Elbow 2020;0(0):1–7.

38. Sheth U, Saltzman M. Reverse total shoulder arthroplasty: implant design considerations. Curr Rev Musculoskelet Med 2019;12:554–61.

39. Werner BS, Ascione F, Bugelli G, et al. Does arm lengthening affect the functional outcome in onlay reverse shoulder arthroplasty? J Shoulder Elbow Surg 2017;26:2152–7.

40. Haidamous G, Lädermann A, Frankle MA, et al. The risk of postoperative scapular spine fracture following reverse shoulder arthroplasty is increased with an onlay humeral stem. J Shoulder Elbow Surg 2020;29:2556–63.

41. Wong MT, Langohr DG, Athwal GS, et al. Implant positioning in reverse shoulder arthroplasty has an impact on acromial stresses. J Shoulder Elbow Surg 2016;25:1889–95.

42. Matsen FA III, Boileau P, Walch G, et al. The reverse total shoulder arthroplasty. J Bone Joint Surg Am. 2007;89(3):660–7.

43. Farshad M, Gerber C. Reverse total shoulder arthroplasty-from the most to the least common complications. Int Orthop 2010;34:1075–82.

44. Mayne IP, Bell SN, Wright W, et al. Acromial and scapular spine fractures after reverse total shoulder arthroplasty. Shoulder Elbow 2016;8:90–100.

45. Wahlquist TC, Hunt AF, Braman JP. Acromial base fractures after reverse total shoulder arthroplasty: report of five cases. J Shoulder Elbow Surg 2011; 20:1178–83.

Complications After Anatomic Shoulder Arthroplasty

Revisiting Leading Causes of Failure

Paul J. Weatherby, MD[a], Tsola A. Efejuku, BSA[b],
Jeremy S. Somerson, MD[a],*

KEYWORDS

- Anatomic • Shoulder arthroplasty • Replacement • Complications • Failure • Loosening
- Glenoid • Rotator cuff

KEY POINTS

- With advances in implant design and techniques, the complication profile after anatomic shoulder arthroplasty is changing and outcomes are improving.
- Recent published evidence and database reports show a decline in the relative rate of glenoid loosening, while rotator cuff insufficiency remains common.
- Understanding the factors that have led to improved outcomes can help surgeons reduce their risk of postoperative complications.

INTRODUCTION

Anatomic total shoulder arthroplasty (aTSA) has become a frequently performed procedure across the United States, with the annual number of shoulder arthroplasties demonstrating a fivefold increase between 2000 and 2010.[1] This trend has continued over the past decade, from 9.5 cases per 100,000 to 12.5 cases per 100,000 annually from 2012 to 2017.[2] The future growth of shoulder arthroplasty is expected to outpace the growth in total hip and knee arthroplasty.[3] With this dramatic increase in procedures performed, there is increasing interest in exploring the complications associated with this surgery.

A prior review of anatomic shoulder arthroplasty literature attributed more than a third of reported complications to glenoid component loosening (37% of complications); substantially lower relative percentages of complications were attributed to rotator cuff failure (9%) and humeral loosening (1%).[4] These data were derived from published outcomes in 33 studies, with a mean of more than 100 reported shoulder arthroplasties per study. However, most shoulder arthroplasty procedures are performed by surgeons with substantially lower clinical volume. In a review of a major integrated health system's arthroplasty database in 2010, approximately one-third of shoulder arthroplasty procedures were performed by surgeons performing a median of 3 to 4 shoulder arthroplasties per year.[5] Surgeon experience has also been shown to affect the complication profile after shoulder arthroplasty. Recent Australian registry data have shown a significantly different complication profile for lower-volume surgeons.[6]

With this background, it is unlikely that published series of shoulder arthroplasty outcomes

---

The authors received no financial support for the research, authorship, and/or publication of this article.
^a Department of Orthopaedic Surgery and Rehabilitation, The University of Texas Medical Branch, 301 University Boulevard, Galveston, TX 77555, USA; ^b School of Medicine, The University of Texas Medical Branch, 301 University Boulevard, Galveston, TX 77555, USA
* Corresponding author.
E-mail address: jeremysomerson@gmail.com

from high-volume centers accurately reflect the complications that occur in current practice. In this work, we review a broader range of sources, including registry reports and a US Food and Drug Administration (FDA) database, to revisit the leading causes of failure after aTSA. We also review technical, design, and patient-selection factors that may reduce complications.

Glenoid Component Failure

Glenoid component loosening is described in the literature as the leading cause of failure of total shoulder arthroplasties.[7-11] In 1997, Torchia and colleagues[11] reported results as high as 82% of radiolucency at the bone-cement interface and 11% of radiographic glenoid component loosening with a 10-year follow-up. Bohsali and colleagues[4] analyzed 33 studies with 3360 shoulders (345 complications) and found glenoid component loosening to comprise 37.7% of all reported failures.

Although glenoid component failure continues to be common after shoulder arthroplasty, recent data show this to be a smaller percentage of all complications than previously reported. A review of the FDA's Manufacturer and User Facility Device Experience (MAUDE) database of medical device complications showed that glenoid component loosening comprised 20.4% (341 of 1673 adverse events) of all complications related to anatomic shoulder arthroplasty devices.[12] Similar findings have been noted in registry reports. A recent review of the Australian Orthopedic Association National Joint Replacement Registry 2020 showed that implant loosening was the reason for revision in only 18% of cases (208 of 1182 revisions), compared with 26% of revisions due to rotator cuff insufficiency and 22% due to instability.[13] Despite severe radiographic findings, many cases of radiographic glenoid loosening may be clinically asymptomatic. For example, a patient with severe osteolysis around a pegged glenoid implant (Fig. 1) had a stable clinical outcome at more than 5 years and did not undergo revision surgery.

Management of posterior glenoid bone loss

One potential explanation for the relative decrease in the observed rates of glenoid loosening is the use of specific techniques to manage posterior glenoid bone loss and biconcavity. In the past, a technique of substantial eccentric reaming of the anterior glenoid was frequently used to alter glenoid version in severely retroverted cases.[14,15] This resulted in a high rate of glenoid loosening, leading to recommendations that this technique should be limited to correct only 10° to 15° of retroversion.[16] However, a recent study of computed tomography scans in arthritic shoulders with posterior wear showed that even small amounts of eccentric reaming and version correction resulted in significant losses in glenoid bone density.[17]

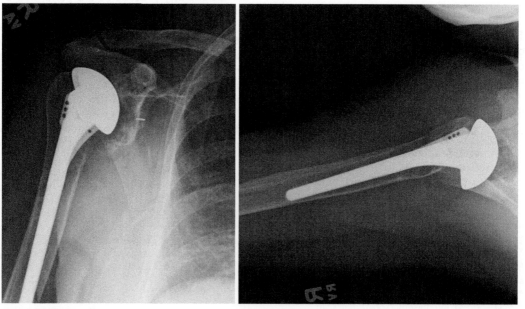

Fig. 1. Anteroposterior and lateral radiographs of a right shoulder showing high-grade osteolysis and formation of radiolucent lines. The patient reported a good functional outcome despite these radiographic changes.

Alternative approaches have shown successful early outcomes. Matsen and colleagues[18] reported outcomes with minimal reaming of eccentric glenoids without any attempt to alter glenoid retroversion (Fig. 2). Of the 156 patients with a B1, B2, or B3-type eccentric glenoid, only 2 patients showed osteolysis at the central peg at minimum 2-year follow-up (1.3%) and no glenoid revisions were performed. A prior study by this group showed no difference in 2-year minimum radiographic or clinical outcomes with glenoid components implanted in 15° or more of retroversion, compared with glenoid implants with less than 15° of retroversion.[19] In this study, 29% of shoulders with a retroverted glenoid implant showed radiolucent lines, none of which

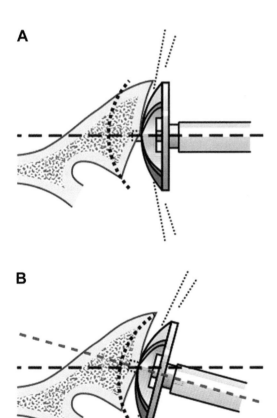

Fig. 2. Comparison of (A) eccentric reaming in an effort to correct version and (B) noncorrective reaming. A substantially greater portion of supportive subchondral bone is lost with corrective reaming. (*From* Matsen FA 3rd, Lippitt SB, Rockwood CA Jr, Wirth MA. Glenohumeral arthritis and its management. *Rockwood and Matsen's The Shoulder*, 5th Edition. 2016: 831-1042; with permission.)

were greater than Lazarus grade 2. Longer-term study is necessary to determine whether these results are stable at mid-term and long-term follow-up.

Posteriorly augmented glenoid components have also shown promising early clinical results for treatment of posterior glenoid bone loss. Grey and colleagues[20] reported the minimum 2-year outcomes of 68 patients undergoing anatomic shoulder arthroplasty using an 8-degree posteriorly augmented glenoid. Two patients (3%) had undergone glenoid component revision at a minimum of 2 years. Just over one-third of patients (21 of 57 patients, 37%) were observed to have formation of radiolucent lines on postoperative radiographs. Similar findings were reported by Priddy and colleagues,[21] with 37 patients undergoing anatomic shoulder arthroplasty with posteriorly augmented full-wedge glenoid components. Patients showed significant improvement in patient-reported outcomes. There were 2 revision surgeries (5%), only 1 of which was for glenoid loosening. Radiolucent lines were noted in 54% of patients at final follow-up, with 22% showing more severe Lazarus grade 4 or 5 changes. The clinical significance of these early radiolucencies is unknown but warrants longer-term observation.

Some investigators have proposed the use of reverse TSA (rTSA) for patients with an intact rotator cuff, but eccentric glenoid wear and posterior bone loss. Mizuno and colleagues[22] reported 27 cases of rTSA performed for primary glenohumeral arthritis in the setting of a biconcave glenoid. At a minimum of 2 years, 1 shoulder (4%) showed loosening of the glenoid component, and 10 shoulders (37%) had visible scapular notching. McFarland and colleagues[23] reported similar outcomes among 42 patients with severe glenoid wear and an intact rotator cuff who underwent shoulder arthroplasty. Significant improvements were noted in all patient-reported outcome measures, with 1 revision surgery (2%) due to baseplate failure and 8 shoulders (19%) with radiographic evidence of notching. Although prior studies have shown deterioration in long-term outcomes at 10 years after rTSA,[24] it is unclear whether patients with an intact rotator cuff will have a similar long-term decline.

Use of cemented all-polyethylene glenoid components

There has been increasing use of cross-linked, all-polyethylene, cemented glenoid components,[25–27] all of which have been associated with lower revision rates compared with non–cross-linked, metal-backed, and uncemented components (Table 1). A randomized controlled trial by Boileau and colleagues[28] raised early concerns about the use of metal-backed glenoids, with clear evidence that cementless, metal-backed glenoid components had a high rate of failure. These results were echoed by case series from high-volume centers showing higher-than-expected rates of revision.[29–31] Despite this, many groups continued to pursue the use of metal-backed uncemented components. A systematic review published in 2014 identified 21 studies reporting outcomes for 1571 shoulder arthroplasties using a metal-backed glenoid.[32] The rate of revision was 14% in the metal-backed glenoid group, compared with 4% for a comparable group of all-polyethylene glenoids. The investigators postulated that the increased failure rate was due to the increased thickness of the metal-backed components resulting in joint line lateralization and material stiffness mismatches among bone, metal, and polyethylene.

Pegged versus keeled glenoid implants

Most long-term studies of aTSA report the outcomes of keeled glenoid implants.[33–35] After publication of a randomized controlled trial in 2010 demonstrating superior outcomes for a pegged glenoid design,[36] many manufacturers adopted a pegged glenoid component. A recent systematic review showed a lower revision rate with pegged implant designs compared with keeled designs, although no significant differences were noted with respect to functional outcomes.[37] It is unclear whether the radiolucent lines noted in short-term studies of pegged implants[38,39] will result in similar long-term declines as those noted for keeled implants.

Rotator Cuff Insufficiency

Historically, rotator cuff insufficiency after aTSA has represented less than 10% of published complications.[4] However, there has been a relative increase in reported rates of this complication. A large, international, multicenter study group recently reported that rotator cuff tears were the most common complication after 2224 aTSA procedures, with an incidence of 3.1% and comprising a relative 28.9% of all complications.[40] Higher rates of rotator cuff dysfunction have been reported in longer-term studies. Young and colleagues[41] studied 518 shoulders and noted a 17% rate of rotator cuff dysfunction at a mean follow-up of 8.6 years. They defined "dysfunction" as greater than 25% superior migration of the humeral component on a true anteroposterior radiograph of the glenohumeral joint; factors that increased risk of rotator cuff tears in their study were duration of follow-up, superior tilt of the glenoid component, and infraspinatus atrophy. Furthermore, Levy and colleagues[42] in 2016 performed a systematic review of 15 studies (1338 shoulders) and reported a nearly 30% rate of radiographic superior migration.

There is limited evidence to identify risk factors for secondary rotator cuff failure after aTSA. In a retrospective study of minimum 2-year outcomes, Choate and colleagues[43] found that preoperative partial thickness supraspinatus tears and positive tangent signs did not correlate with postoperative objective range of motion or patient-reported outcomes. Levy and colleagues[42] identified inadequate subscapularis repair, humeral component malrotation, oversized components, glenoid and/or capsular deficiency and deltoid deficiency as risk factors for subscapularis failure and anterior instability. Fig. 3 demonstrates a patient who underwent

Table 1
Technical factors associated with glenoid revision rates in the Australian Orthopedic Association National Joint Replacement Registry

Factor	
Cementless glenoid fixation	Higher rate of revision compared with cemented glenoid fixation
Use of metal-backed glenoid components	Higher rate of revision compared with all-polyethylene glenoid components
Use of cross-linked polyethylene (XLPE) glenoids	Lower cumulative rate of revision at 10 y compared with non-XLPE glenoids

Data from Australian Orthopaedic Association National Joint Replacement Registry (AOANJRR). Hip, Knee & Shoulder Arthroplasty Annual Report, AOA, Adelaide; 2020. Available at: https://aoanjrr.sahmri.com/annual-reports-2020. Accessed December 9, 2020.

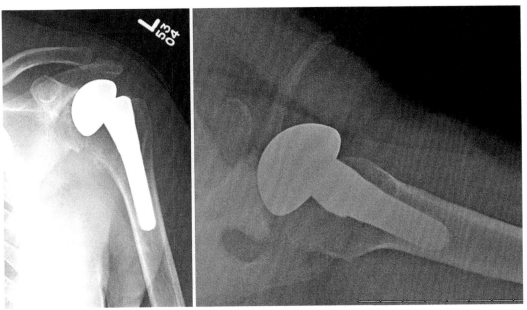

Fig. 3. Anteroposterior and axillary lateral views of a humeral hemiarthroplasty extending well superior to the greater tuberosity. At the time of revision to reverse shoulder arthroplasty, the rotator cuff was found to be torn and retracted.

hemiarthroplasty with oversized and proud humeral components. At the time of revision surgery, the supraspinatus was found to be torn and retracted. The patient was revised to rTSA with a good clinical outcome. Patient compliance with restrictions is also an important factor to consider. **Fig. 4** demonstrates evidence of subscapularis failure in a patient who felt increased pain after lifting a heavy box 8 weeks after aTSA. At 14 weeks postoperatively, the patient returned for follow-up and underwent revision surgery. The prosthesis was converted to rTSA (see **Fig. 4**) after the subscapularis was found to be insufficient for repair.

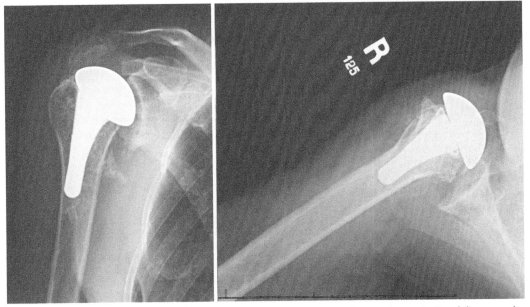

Fig. 4. Anteroposterior and axillary lateral views of a total shoulder arthroplasty with anterior instability secondary to subscapularis rupture. At the time of revision, the subscapularis was found to be irreparable. The prosthesis was revised to a reverse shoulder arthroplasty.

Painful Arthroplasty Without Identifiable Etiology

A painful or stiff arthroplasty without an identifiable etiology is uncommonly reported in published literature, but was the third-most prominent among failure modes in the FDA MAUDE database (215 patients, 12.9%).[12] Although some of these patients likely had other unrecognized etiologies, such as low-grade infection, practicing arthroplasty surgeons will be familiar with this small subset of patients who continue to have pain despite careful exclusion of infection, rotator cuff pathology, and loosening. Thompson and colleagues[44] noted that patients who were taking narcotic pain medication for at least 3 months before surgery had inferior American Shoulder and Elbow Surgeons scores and visual analog scale scores when compared with non-narcotic patients. This same subset of patients had less forward elevation, external rotation, and all strength measurements. They concluded that chronic preoperative narcotic use might be an indicator of poor outcomes in anatomic total shoulder replacement. In addition, Wells and colleagues[45] performed a retrospective review of patients who were current tobacco users, former tobacco users, and nonusers in the setting of aTSA. They found mean improvement in visual analog scores of tobacco users was significantly lower than in nonusers and former tobacco users.

DISCUSSION

Recent literature suggests that the complication profile after aTSA is changing. This may be due to a gradual refinement of techniques and implant choices. A systematic review of shoulder arthroplasty literature between 1990 and 2015 showed steady improvement in clinical outcomes after anatomic shoulder arthroplasty.[46] This improvement in outcomes was also seen in the Norwegian Arthroplasty Register, in which anatomic total shoulders showed markedly improved 5-year survival rates from 1994 to 2012.[47]

Glenoid loosening has shown a decrease in overall rates over the past 3 decades. Widespread usage of an all-polyethylene cemented glenoid component and evidence-based techniques for management of the B2 glenoid are likely contributors to this. In addition, many patients with rotator cuff insufficiency, severe glenoid wear, or posttraumatic pathology are now more commonly treated with reverse TSA.

In contrast, registry data, recent case series, and the FDA MAUDE database have shown other failure modes to be more prevalent than previously reported (Table 2). Revision for rotator cuff insufficiency may now be the most common current reason for revision after anatomic TSA.

Table 2
Complications as a percentage of all reported complications after anatomic arthroplasty, as published in 3 sources

Data Source Number of Complications Type of Source Complication Type	Bohsali et al[a] [N = 345] Systematic Review %	MAUDE[b] [N = 1673] FDA Database %	AOANJRR 2020[c] [N = 1182] National Registry %
Component loosening	39	25	18
Instability	10	12	22
Rotator cuff insufficiency	9	15	26
Infection	5	9	7
Pain/stiffness	Unknown	13	4

Abbreviations: AOANJRR, Australian Orthopedic Association National Joint Replacement Registry; FDA, Food and Drug Administration; MAUDE, Manufacturer and User Facility Device Experience.

[a] Data from: A systematic review of published complications after shoulder arthroplasty. Bohsali KI., Bois AJ., Wirth MA. Complications of Shoulder Arthroplasty: The Journal of Bone and Joint Surgery 2017;99(3):256–69.

[b] Data from: An analysis of the FDA Manufacturer and User Facility Device Experience (MAUDE) database. Somerson JS., Hsu JE., Neradilek MB., et al. Analysis of 4063 complications of shoulder arthroplasty reported to the US Food and Drug Administration from 2012 to 2016. J Shoulder Elbow Surg 2018;27(11):1978–86.

[c] Data from: Australian Orthopaedic Association National Joint Replacement Registry. Hip, Knee & Shoulder Arthroplasty Annual Report, AOA, Adelaide; 2020. Available at: https://aoanjrr.sahmri.com/annual-reports-2020. Accessed December 9, 2020.

One potential contributor to this is increasing surgeon experience with reverse TSA for revision in cases of rotator cuff failure.[48] Avoidance of oversized components, meticulous subscapularis repair, and counseling of patients regarding postoperative limitations may be beneficial in avoiding this growing source of complications. Careful patient selection regarding preoperative nicotine and opioid use may also reduce the risks of a painful arthroplasty without a recognized etiology.

One limitation of reviewing complications and failures is that definitions of a complication may vary substantially. Registry data and the MAUDE database typically report only revision surgeries, whereas published literature is more likely to report failure modes that do not result in revision. This may contribute to the decreased rate of glenoid loosening observed in registry data and the MAUDE database, as early stages of glenoid loosening are often asymptomatic and treated with observation.

For practicing surgeons, it is advisable to consider a breadth of data sources concerning complications and outcomes. Although published series from high-volume centers are the primary source of data, these results may not be generalizable to a wide range of practice settings because of disparities in experience and patient populations.[49] The FDA MAUDE database is publicly available[50] and can be searched by manufacturer, product name, and type of implant. National or health system–specific registry databases are also useful to assess the changing complication profile of shoulder arthroplasty, as well as to understand the complications specific to certain implants or implant types.[51] To reduce the risk of postoperative complications, surgeons must have a clear understanding of the most common modes of failure.

CLINICS CARE POINTS

- Use of a cemented, all-polyethylene glenoid component has led to a reduction in rates of revision for glenoid loosening over time.
- Management of posterior glenoid wear and biconcavity with eccentric reaming reduces the strength of subchondral bone and has been associated with increased formation of radiolucencies.
- Alternatives to eccentric reaming include noncorrective reaming with acceptance of implant retroversion, augmented glenoid components or rTSA.

- Current literature demonstrates that the relative rates of rotator cuff failure/instability and painful/stiff arthroplasty without identifiable cause are increasing.
- Strategies to avoid secondary rotator cuff insufficiency after aTSA include meticulous subscapularis repair, avoidance of oversized or proud implants, and clear communication with patients about postoperative limitations.
- Chronic pain after arthroplasty is associated with preoperative nicotine and opioid use.

ACKNOWLEDGMENTS

The authors thank Jennifer Edwards for her invaluable assistance with editing this article.

DISCLOSURE

J.S. Somerson has received support for educational programs from Medinc of Texas, Skeletal Dynamics, Bioventus, Amgen, Smith and Nephew, and ConvaTec. The other authors have nothing to disclose.

REFERENCES

1. Trofa D, Rajaee SS, Smith EL. Nationwide trends in total shoulder arthroplasty and hemiarthroplasty for osteoarthritis. Am J Orthop (Belle Mead NJ) 2014;43(4):166–72.
2. Best MJ, Aziz KT, Wilckens JH, et al. Increasing incidence of primary reverse and anatomic total shoulder arthroplasty in the United States. J Shoulder Elbow Surg 2020. https://doi.org/10.1016/j.jse.2020.08.010.
3. Wagner ER, Farley KX, Higgins I, et al. The incidence of shoulder arthroplasty: rise and future projections compared with hip and knee arthroplasty. J Shoulder Elbow Surg 2020;29(12):2601–9.
4. Bohsali KI, Bois AJ, Wirth MA. Complications of shoulder arthroplasty. J Bone Joint Surg 2017; 99(3):256–69.
5. Singh A, Yian EH, Dillon MT, et al. The effect of surgeon and hospital volume on shoulder arthroplasty perioperative quality metrics. J Shoulder Elbow Surg 2014;23(8):1187–94.
6. Brown JS, Gordon RJ, Peng Y, et al. Lower operating volume in shoulder arthroplasty is associated with increased revision rates in the early postoperative period: long-term analysis from the Australian Orthopaedic Association National Joint Replacement Registry. J Shoulder Elbow Surg 2020;29(6): 1104–14.
7. Walch G, Young AA, Boileau P, et al. Patterns of loosening of polyethylene keeled glenoid components after shoulder arthroplasty for primary

osteoarthritis: results of a multicenter study with more than five years of follow-up. J Bone Joint Surg 2012;94(2):145–50.

8. Franklin JL, Barrett WP, Jackins SE, et al. Glenoid loosening in total shoulder arthroplasty. Association with rotator cuff deficiency. J Arthroplasty 1988;3(1):39–46.

9. Fox TJ, Cil A, Sperling JW, et al. Survival of the glenoid component in shoulder arthroplasty. J Shoulder Elbow Surg 2009;18(6):859–63.

10. Papadonikolakis A, Neradilek MB, Matsen I Frederick A. Failure of the glenoid component in anatomic total shoulder arthroplastya systematic review of the English-language literature between 2006 and 2012. J Bone Joint Surg 2013;95(24):2205–12.

11. Torchia ME, Cofield RH, Settergren CR. Total shoulder arthroplasty with the neer prosthesis: long-term results. J Shoulder Elbow Surg 1997;6(6):495–505.

12. Somerson JS, Hsu JE, Neradilek MB, et al. Analysis of 4063 complications of shoulder arthroplasty reported to the US Food and Drug Administration from 2012 to 2016. J Shoulder Elbow Surg 2018;27(11):1978–86.

13. Australian Orthopaedic Association National Joint Replacement Registry (AOANJRR). Hip, Knee & Shoulder Arthroplasty Annual Report, AOA, Adelaide. 2020. Available at: https://aoanjrr.sahmri.com/annual-reports-2020. Accessed December 9, 2020.

14. Walch G, Moraga C, Young A, et al. Results of anatomic nonconstrained prosthesis in primary osteoarthritis with biconcave glenoid. J Shoulder Elbow Surg 2012;21(11):1526–33.

15. Ho JC, Sabesan VJ, Iannotti JP. Glenoid component retroversion is associated with osteolysis. J Bone Joint Surg Am 2013;95(12):e82.

16. Stephens SP, Paisley KC, Jeng J, et al. Shoulder arthroplasty in the presence of posterior glenoid bone loss. J Bone Joint Surg 2015;97(3):251–9.

17. Chen X, Reddy AS, Kontaxis A, et al. Version correction via eccentric reaming compromises remaining bone quality in b2 glenoids: a computational study. Clin Orthop Relat Res 2017;475(12):3090–9.

18. Matsen FAI, Whitson AJ, Somerson JS, et al. Anatomic total shoulder arthroplasty with all-polyethylene glenoid component for primary osteoarthritis with glenoid deficiencies. JBJS Open Access 2020;5(4). e20.00002.

19. Service BC, Hsu JE, Somerson JS, et al. Does postoperative glenoid retroversion affect the 2-year clinical and radiographic outcomes for total shoulder arthroplasty? Clin Orthop 2017;475(11):2726–39.

20. Grey SG, Wright TW, Flurin P-H, et al. Clinical and radiographic outcomes with a posteriorly augmented glenoid for Walch B glenoids in anatomic total shoulder arthroplasty. J Shoulder Elbow Surg 2020;29(5):e185–95.

21. Priddy M, Zarezadeh A, Farmer KW, et al. Early results of augmented anatomic glenoid components. J Shoulder Elbow Surg 2019;28(6, Supplement):S138–45.

22. Mizuno N, Denard PJ, Raiss P, et al. Reverse total shoulder arthroplasty for primary glenohumeral osteoarthritis in patients with a biconcave glenoid. JBJS 2013;95(14):1297–304.

23. McFarland EG, Huri G, Hyun YS, et al. Reverse total shoulder arthroplasty without bone-grafting for severe glenoid bone loss in patients with osteoarthritis and intact rotator cuff. J Bone Joint Surg Am 2016;98(21):1801–7.

24. Bacle G, Nové-Josserand L, Garaud P, et al. Long-term outcomes of reverse total shoulder arthroplasty: a follow-up of a previous study. JBJS 2017;99(6):454–61.

25. Sharplin PK, Frampton CMA, Hirner M. Cemented vs. uncemented glenoid fixation in total shoulder arthroplasty for osteoarthritis: a New Zealand Joint Registry study. J Shoulder Elbow Surg 2020;29(10):2097–103.

26. Page RS, Pai V, Eng K, et al. Cementless versus cemented glenoid components in conventional total shoulder joint arthroplasty: analysis from the Australian Orthopaedic Association National Joint Replacement Registry. J Shoulder Elbow Surg 2018;27(10):1859–65.

27. Matsen FA, Iannotti JP, Churchill RS, et al. One and two-year clinical outcomes for a polyethylene glenoid with a fluted peg: one thousand two hundred seventy individual patients from eleven centers. Int Orthop 2019;43(2):367–78.

28. Boileau P, Avidor C, Krishnan SG, et al. Cemented polyethylene versus uncemented metal-backed glenoid components in total shoulder arthroplasty: A prospective, double-blind, randomized study. J Shoulder Elbow Surg 2002;11(4):351–9.

29. Taunton MJ, McIntosh AL, Sperling JW, et al. Total shoulder arthroplasty with a metal-backed, bone-ingrowth glenoid componentmedium to long-term results. J Bone Joint Surg 2008;90(10):2180–8.

30. Fucentese SF, Costouros JG, Kühnel S-P, et al. Total shoulder arthroplasty with an uncemented soft-metal-backed glenoid component. J Shoulder Elbow Surg 2010;19(4):624–31.

31. Gauci MO, Bonnevialle N, Moineau G, et al. Anatomical total shoulder arthroplasty in young patients with osteoarthritis: all-polyethylene versus metal-backed glenoid. Bone Joint J 2018;100-B(4):485–92.

32. Papadonikolakis A, Matsen FA. Metal-backed glenoid components have a higher rate of failure and fail by different modes in comparison with

all-polyethylene components. J Bone Joint Surg Am 2014;96(12):1041–7.

33. Raiss P, Bruckner T, Rickert M, et al. Longitudinal observational study of total shoulder replacements with cement: fifteen to twenty-year follow-up. J Bone Joint Surg 2014;96(3):198–205.

34. Denard PJ, Raiss P, Sowa B, et al. Mid- to long-term follow-up of total shoulder arthroplasty using a keeled glenoid in young adults with primary glenohumeral arthritis. J Shoulder Elbow Surg 2013;22(7): 894–900.

35. Schoch BS., Sperling JW., Cofield RH., et al. Minimum 20-year follow up of Neer shoulder arthroplasty in patients less than 50 years. American Academy of Orthopaedic Surgeons 2014 Annual Meeting. New Orleans: March 11–15, 2014 n.d.

36. Edwards TB, Labriola JE, Stanley RJ, et al. Radiographic comparison of pegged and keeled glenoid components using modern cementing techniques: a prospective randomized study. J Shoulder Elbow Surg 2010;19(2):251–7.

37. Welsher A, Gohal C, Madden K, et al. A comparison of pegged vs. keeled glenoid components regarding functional and radiographic outcomes in anatomic total shoulder arthroplasty: a systematic review and meta-analysis. JSES Open Access 2019;3(3):136–44.e1.

38. Wijeratna M, Taylor DM, Lee S, et al. Clinical and radiographic results of an all-polyethylene pegged bone-ingrowth glenoid component. J Bone Joint Surg Am 2016;98(13):1090–6.

39. Merolla G, Ciaramella G, Fabbri E, et al. Total shoulder replacement using a bone ingrowth central peg polyethylene glenoid component: a prospective clinical and computed tomography study with short- to mid-term follow-up. Int Orthop 2016;40(11):2355–63.

40. Parada SA, Flurin P-H, Wright TW, et al. Comparison of complication types and rates associated with anatomic and reverse total shoulder arthroplasty. J Shoulder Elbow Surg 2020. https://doi.org/10.1016/j.jse.2020.07.028.

41. Young AA, Walch G, Pape G, et al. Secondary rotator cuff dysfunction following total shoulder arthroplasty for primary glenohumeral osteoarthritis: results of a multicenter study with more than five years of follow-up. J Bone Joint Surg Am 2012; 94(8):685–93.

42. Levy DM, Abrams GD, Harris JD, et al. Rotator cuff tears after total shoulder arthroplasty in primary osteoarthritis: a systematic review. Int J Shoulder Surg 2016;10(2):78–84.

43. Choate WS, Shanley E, Washburn R, et al. The incidence and effect of fatty atrophy, positive tangent sign, and rotator cuff tears on outcomes after total shoulder arthroplasty. J Shoulder Elbow Surg 2017; 26(12):2110–6.

44. Thompson KM, Hallock JD, Smith RA, et al. Preoperative narcotic use and inferior outcomes after anatomic total shoulder arthroplasty: a clinical and radiographic analysis. J Am Acad Orthop Surg 2019;27(5):177–82.

45. Wells DB, Holt AM, Smith RA, et al. Tobacco use predicts a more difficult episode of care after anatomic total shoulder arthroplasty. J Shoulder Elbow Surg 2018;27(1):23–8.

46. Somerson JS, Neradilek MB, Hsu JE, et al. Is there evidence that the outcomes of primary anatomic and reverse shoulder arthroplasty are getting better? Int Orthop 2017;41(6):1235–44.

47. Fevang BTS, Nystad TW, Skredderstuen A, et al. Improved survival for anatomic total shoulder prostheses. Acta Orthop 2015;86(1):63–70.

48. Sheth MM, Sholder D, Getz CL, et al. Revision of failed hemiarthroplasty and anatomic total shoulder arthroplasty to reverse total shoulder arthroplasty. J Shoulder Elbow Surg 2019;28(6):1074–81.

49. Somerson JS, Stein BA, Wirth MA. Distribution of high-volume shoulder arthroplasty surgeons in the United States: data from the 2014 medicare provider utilization and payment data release. J Bone Joint Surg Am 2016;98(18):e77.

50. MAUDE - Manufacturer and User Facility Device Experience. Available at: https://www.accessdata.fda.gov/scripts/cdrh/cfdocs/cfMAUDE/search.CFM. Accessed May 16, 2017.

51. Bayona CEA, Somerson JS, Matsen FA. The utility of international shoulder joint replacement registries and databases: a comparative analytic review of two hundred and sixty one thousand, four hundred and eighty four cases. Int Orthop 2018;42(2): 351–8.

Foot and Ankle

Complications Associated with Peripheral Nerve Blocks

Kevin H. Phan, MD*, John G. Anderson, MD,
Donald R. Bohay, MD, FACS

KEYWORDS

- Peripheral • Nerve • Block • Complications • Foot • Ankle • Surgery

KEY POINTS

- Peripheral nerve blocks are becoming standard of care in foot and ankle surgery for their effectiveness and low complication rates.
- The most common complication of peripheral nerve blocks is peripheral nerve injury, which can be caused by mechanical trauma, neurotoxic trauma, or ischemic trauma to the nerve.
- Preoperative discussion with patients should include potential complications from the nerve block.

INTRODUCTION

Regional anesthesia in the form of peripheral nerve blocks (PNBs) is quickly becoming the gold standard in perioperative pain management, not only in foot and ankle surgery but also for all of orthopedics.[1–7] There has been a push toward outpatient surgery in the recent years in an attempt to cut down on hospital costs.[8,9] PNBs provide excellent perioperative pain relief during the first 24 hours after surgery, which are generally the most painful, allowing patients to be discharged immediately after surgery. A study by Hadzic and colleagues[3] showed that patients undergoing outpatient knee surgery who received PNBs more often bypassed the higher level of care recovery unit, phase I Postanesthesia Care Unit (PACU), and had less postoperative nausea and vomiting than patients given general anesthesia. Less side effects from heavy doses of general anesthetic leads to expedited discharges home and improved patient satisfaction.[3,10] PNBs are also effective in reducing patient opioid requirements,[11] which is especially relevant during these times, as

orthopedic surgeons are dealing with the opioid crisis.[12,13]

As PNBs become more and more widely used in both hospital and outpatient settings, new techniques have been developed in order to make the procedure as safe as possible for patients and to maximize its efficacy.[14] Nerve stimulation and ultrasound-guided techniques are used in order to ensure that anesthetic medication is not injected directly into major nerves or blood vessels, which can cause significant morbidity and even mortality. However, the most common complication from PNBs is neuropathic symptoms. It has been reported that patients experience long-term symptoms in less than 1% of patients,[15–18] but some studies have found residual neuropathic symptoms in up to 24% of patients at 8 months postoperatively.[19–21] For the most part, these symptoms tend to spontaneously resolve within days to weeks[22]; however, symptoms have been found to last up to 8 months after surgery.[20] A less common complication, but with more severe consequences, is local anesthetic systemic toxicity (LAST), when local anesthetic is injected

Orthopaedic Associates of Michigan, 1111 Leffingwell Avenue Northeast, Grand Rapids, MI 49525, USA
* Corresponding author.
E-mail address: kevinphan87@gmail.com

intravascularly, which can be a life-threatening event.[23]

It is important to understand the risks involved with PNBs as they become more and more widely used, not only to try to minimize the risks to patients but also to better inform patients about the possible adverse effects from surgery.

BACKGROUND
Anatomy of Nerves Supplying the Foot and Ankle

Sensation in the foot and ankle is supplied by the saphenous, tibial, superficial peroneal, and deep peroneal nerves. The saphenous nerve is a branch of the femoral nerve, whereas the others are distal branches of the sciatic nerve. The saphenous nerve supplies sensation to the medial aspect of the foot and ankle. The tibial nerve provides sensation to the plantar foot via the medial and lateral plantar nerves. The superficial peroneal nerve provides sensation to the dorsum of the foot, and the deep peroneal nerve provides sensation to the first web space. The sural nerve provides sensation to the lateral aspect of the posterior ankle and foot and originates from branches of the tibial and common peroneal nerves.

Popliteal Nerve Block

The popliteal block is widely used, as it is easy to visualize on ultrasound and targets the sciatic nerve at the level of the popliteal fossa. The goal is to target the sciatic nerve proximal to where it branches into the tibial nerve and common peroneal nerve, which is about 5 to 7 cm proximal to the popliteal crease (**Fig. 1**).[24] An anesthetic administration at this level would provide anesthesia to almost the entire foot and ankle, excluding the medial aspect supplied by the saphenous nerve. Some anatomic landmarks to know and look for are the popliteal artery, which is medial to the sciatic nerve. The sciatic nerve at this level is also bordered medially by the semimembranosus and laterally by the biceps femoris. Inferiorly, the borders are the medial and lateral heads of the gastrocnemius muscle.

Saphenous Nerve Block

This block is performed by injecting anesthetic into the medial aspect of the knee. The saphenous nerve is a pure sensory nerve branch of the femoral nerve and provides sensation to the medial aspect of the foot and ankle. This block in addition to the popliteal nerve block provides complete anesthesia to the foot and

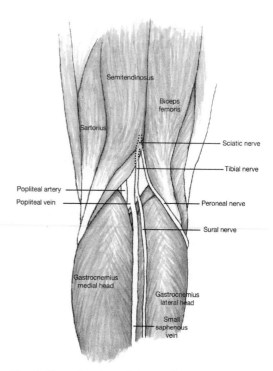

Fig. 1. Posterior view of the popliteal fossa. At this level, the sciatic nerve branches into the common peroneal nerve and the tibial nerve. (*From* Anderson JG, Bohay DR, Maskill JD, et al. Complications after popliteal block for foot and ankle surgery. *Foot Ankle Int.* 2015;36(10):1138-1143. https://doi.org/10.1177/1071100715589741; with permission)

ankle. The nerve can be found in a fascial plane between the vastus medialis and sartorius muscles. At the level of the superior pole of the patella, this fascial plane acts as a landmark for identifying the proper compartment containing the nerve when performing this block using ultrasound.[25]

Peripheral Nerve Blocks Distal to the Knee

These blocks are performed by the surgeon and entails injection of local anesthetic in the perineural region of each nerve in the foot and ankle requiring anesthesia. The technique for this type of block is based on anatomic landmarks. To target the tibial nerve, the surgeon would aim for a spot 2 cm proximal to the medial malleolus and enter perpendicular to the tibial axis and tangential to the medial aspect of the Achilles tendon. The superficial peroneal nerve is anesthetized by injecting subcutaneously across the dorsum of the foot at the level of the ankle. The deep peroneal nerve is targeted by aiming for the deep space in between the first and second metatarsals. The saphenous nerve is targeted with a subcutaneous injection along the anterior aspect of the medial malleolus. The sural nerve is targeted about 1 to 1.5 cm distal to the tip of the fibula.[1,26] Stéfani and colleagues[26] showed that PNBs at the ankle are a safe and effective alternative to the more proximal nerve blocks at the knee. The advantages of these blocks include not needing an anesthesiologist and not needing to perform an ultrasound.

Nerve Localization Techniques
Nerve stimulation versus ultrasound guidance

Ultrasound guidance has all but replaced nerve stimulation as the preferred technique for localizing nerves for regional blocks.[27–30] In the review by Munirama and McLeod[29] of 23 randomized controlled trials (RCTs) comparing nerve stimulation to ultrasound-guided nerve blocks, they found that ultrasound reduced the rate of pain during the procedure, the rate of patients requiring additional anesthesia, and the rate of vascular puncture. Their explanation for this was that owing to patients' varying anatomy, being able to visualize the anatomy before inserting a long needle helps to reduce the rate of injury. It has also been shown that the accepted threshold of nerve stimulation of 0.5 mA may be insufficient to stimulate muscle contraction in up to 25% of patients, resulting in potential intraneural injection.[31] A meta-analysis of 16 RCTs by Gelfand and colleagues[30] showed that ultrasound-guided PNB was associated with a significant increase in the success rate of the block compared with all nonultrasound techniques, including nerve stimulation and utilization of surface landmarks. However, there still has not been a study showing that ultrasound guidance decreases the incidence of peripheral nerve injury (PNI).[32,33] It has, though, significantly decreased the incidence of LAST.[32,34]

Mechanical paresthesia and injection pressure monitoring

Special mention should be made regarding these 2 methods of nerve localization, as they are more subjective than ultrasound guidance or nerve stimulation but are still used. The basis of mechanical paresthesia is that a practitioner would be able to gauge whether his/her needle is intraneural or not based on the patient reporting the sensation of paresthesia or not. There are several issues associated with relying solely on this technique, such as premedication with sedative medication affecting patients'

perception of paresthesia; injection of local anesthetic in the vicinity of the block, which may spread to the peripheral nerve and diminish the impact of any paresthesia produced by needle-nerve contact; and the fact that it has been shown that only 38% of patients experienced paresthesia during needle-nerve contact performed under ultrasound visualization.[31]

The injection pressure monitoring method is based on animal research showing that anesthetic injected at pressures greater than 20 to 25 psi are associated with neurologic dysfunction.[35,36] The basis of this stems from the anatomy of the nerve. Fascicles are composed of thick bundles of nerve fibers, so it makes sense that an intrafascicular injection, which is the most harmful to peripheral nerves,[37] would require more pressure to inject. Lower injection pressures were not associated with nerve injury and seem to indicate extrafascicular injections, which are less harmful to nerves.[35]

Single-Injection Peripheral Nerve Block Versus Continuous Infusion Peripheral Nerve Block

There are 2 types of PNBs that can be used for pain control: single injection and continuous. A single-injection PNB is performed by injecting an anesthetic agent 1 time in the area or areas of interest. A continuous peripheral nerve block (CPNB) is performed by leaving an indwelling catheter connected to a continuous infusion pump, which can deliver a continuous rate of anesthetic over an extended period, usually 2 to 4 days. Single-injection nerve block generally lasts 24 hours postoperatively, whereas CPNBs provide pain relief for about 48 hours postoperatively.[38,39] Patients are generally instructed on how to self-discontinue their catheters on a specified postoperative day. Compared with single PNBs, CPNBs provide significantly better pain relief during the first 3 postoperative days, decreased overall opioid use and therefore less nausea, and greater patient satisfaction.[40,41] Ding and colleagues[42] showed in an RCT of 50 patients with ankle fractures undergoing operative fixation that those who received a CPNB for 48 hours after surgery had significant reductions in rebound pain, need for opioids, and Visual Analogue Scale scores at 2 and 12 weeks. There are however added complications with the CPNB catheters. In the same study, they also reported 8 instances of pump compromise because of catheter dislodgement or pump malfunction. Elliot and colleagues[41] also showed that CPNBs provided a significantly improved pain score; however, the difference in pain scores between CPNB and a single-injection PNB was only between 1.5 and 2 points, which was not clinically significant. Jarrell and colleagues[43] found that using dual nerve catheters in their ambulatory surgical center for foot and ankle surgery yielded better pain control and higher patient satisfaction compared with single nerve catheter with low rates of complications. It is still debatable as to whether the increased pain relief provided by CPNBs is clinically significant enough to warrant the added time required to set up the pump-catheter device as well as educate the patient, the cost of the infusion device, and complications associated with the nerve catheters.

DISCUSSION: COMPLICATIONS

Peripheral Nerve Injury

Long-term PNI is the most commonly reported and feared complication of PNBs because it can lead to significant patient morbidity and dissatisfaction with their surgery. The incidence in the literature is extremely rare (<1%), ranging between 2.4 and 4 per 10,000 blocks.[17,18,32,33,44–47] However, there are reports of rates of residual neurologic symptoms in up to 24% of patients 34 weeks after surgery.[20] Anderson and colleagues[19] have shown a complication rate up to 5% postoperatively in 1014 patients undergoing foot and ankle surgery with popliteal block in an ambulatory setting; the number of long-term complications improved to 0.7% at final follow-up. Fredrickson and Kilfoyle[45] found 8.2% incidence of nerve complication at 10 days postoperatively, which improved to 0.6% at 6 months. In a study by Kahn and colleagues[48] of 2704 foot and ankle procedures that received a PNB, they reported an incidence of block-site complication of 7.2%, with an incidence of serious complication of only 0.7%. The true incidence of PNI is difficult to determine because of the heterogeneity of studies and definitions of PNI in the literature.

Mechanical and injection injury

The mechanisms of PNI fall into 3 categories (Table 1): mechanical and injection, vascular, and chemical.[49] Mechanical-injection injury can be caused by forceful, direct needle-nerve contact or by injection of anesthetic directly into the nerve fascicles.[50] The needle tip punctures the perineurium, which is the outer sheath surrounding the nerve fascicles, allowing injection into the intrafascicular space (Fig. 2), which leads to increased intraneural pressure, which can exceed vascular pressure, causing vascular occlusion and subsequently nerve ischemia.[51] Intrafascicular injections run the highest risk of

Table 1 Peripheral nerve injury	
Mechanical and injection injury	• Direct needle-nerve contact • Intrafascicular injection → leading to increased intraneural pressure → occlusion of neural vasculature • Larger needle gauge causes more damage • Sharper needle bevel more likely to cause damage • Scar tissue resulting from PNB can cause nerve compression
Chemical injury	• All local anesthetics have been found to be neurotoxic • Local anesthetics have also been shown to cause direct vasoconstriction
Vascular injury	• Needle can cause damage to epineurial circulation • Local anesthetics can directly cause vasoconstriction of neural vasculature • Inadvertent intrafascicular injection under high pressure can cause disruption of microvasculature

peripheral nerve axonal degeneration.[37] Therefore, it is imperative for those performing the PNBs to use aids such as ultrasound in order to avoid puncturing the perineurium and directly damaging the nerve fascicles with the needle tip and causing injection trauma. In animal studies, it has been shown that even intrafascicular injections of just saline can cause myelin and axonal degeneration.[37]

The size and shape of the needle also play a role in minimizing the risk of nerve damage during PNBs. Selander and colleagues[52–54] have shown that a needle with a 45° bevel is much less likely to penetrate the perineurium than a needle with a sharper point, such as a 15° bevel; however, the 45° needle, were it to pierce a fascicle, would cause greater damage than if a needle with a 15° bevel were to pierce it. They also showed that the larger the needle gauge, the greater the damage to the nerve after perforation.

Also worth mentioning is the potential compressive effect of scar tissue resulting from

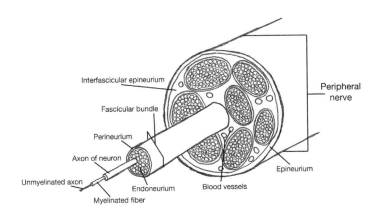

Interfascicular epineurium

Fascicular bundle

Perineurium

Axon of neuron

Unmyelinated axon

Endoneurium   Blood vessels

Myelinated fiber

Peripheral
nerve

Epineurium

Fig. 2. Schematic cross-section of a peripheral nerve, demonstrating the epineurium, perineurium, and endoneurium. Fascicles are tight bundles of nerve fibers that are surrounded by a sheath called the perineurium. (*Courtesy of* L. Behrend, BS, Belmont, MI.)

the inflammation caused by the PNB. Resultant scar tissue in the area can form adhesions and compress peripheral nerves in the vicinity. Kaufman and colleagues[55] have shown this when they surgically explored 14 patients who had chronic diaphragmatic paralysis after an interscalene block. Once the adhesions and scar tissue were taken down, the patients' nerve function was found to improve. There have also been reports from animal data showing that injection of the ultrasound gel itself near nerves can lead to significant intraneural inflammation.[56]

Chemical injury
There is evidence that all local anesthetics are neurotoxic to different degrees.[57–59] The mechanism is thought to be due to an unregulated release of cytosolic calcium, leading to an uncoupling of the oxidative phosphorylation cycle, which ultimately leads to apoptosis.[60–62] There also appears to be a direct correlation between the concentration and duration of exposure of the local anesthetic to the nerve and nerve damage in the form of demyelination, Schwann cell death, and macrophage infiltration.[63,64] Local anesthetics have also been shown to cause direct vasoconstriction, potentially contributing to ischemic nerve injury.[65] Farber and colleagues[59] however showed that even though all commonly used local anesthetics were harmful to some extent, the farther away from the nerve that they were injected, the less damage the nerves sustained. This finding leads us to believe that perhaps what is more important is the proximity of the injection to the nerve rather than the agent itself.

Vascular injury
Decreased blood flow to nerves can cause ischemia and transient or permanent nerve damage. A significant portion, up to 50%, of the

blood supply to a peripheral nerve derives from the epineurial circulation.[66] Damage to this blood supply can result from direct needle trauma or can occur in the presence of an occlusive hematoma.[67,68] In addition, as previously stated, local anesthetics can cause a direct vasoconstriction of the neural vasculature.[65] Inadvertent intrafascicular injection under high pressure could also potentially disrupt the microvasculature.

Risk Factors
There are several patient factors that are out of the health care provider's control that can contribute to a higher likelihood of a perioperative PNB complication. These factors are important to be aware of in order to better counsel patients before surgery.

Age
In a retrospective study conducted by Lauf and colleagues[69] of 855 blocks given for foot and ankle surgery, they found that those patients between the ages of 40 and 65, normal or underweight body mass index (BMI), who underwent surgery at an ambulatory surgical center and who were current smokers had a significantly higher odds ratio of sustaining a perioperative nerve complication. Anderson and colleagues[19] also found that postoperative symptoms were significantly associated with age, as the average age of their patients who had postoperative nerve symptoms was 47.3 years, although they also reported that the average age of patients without symptoms was 50.2 years. At this time, it is unclear why patients within this age range would have higher complications rates.

Body mass index
It is surprising that those of normal or underweight BMI would have a higher odds ratio of nerve damage. Nielsen and colleagues[70] looked

at 9038 nerve blocks performed at an ambulatory surgical center and found that the block failure rate and complication rate were significantly higher in obese patients when compared with nonobese patients. They attributed this to difficulty in proper patient positioning, appropriate landmark identification, and appropriate equipment, such as extralong needles and ultrasound or fluoroscopic guidance. It has been postulated that in patients with less adipose tissue, even though it is easier to visualize anatomy, there is less fatty padding around the nerves to protect it from potential mechanical damage as well as less tissue to absorb excessive anesthetic that could be neurotoxic.[57–59,69]

Smoking

Smoking has been shown to be a significant predictor of postoperative PNB complications.[20,69] There are several proposed mechanisms. One is that the chronic nicotine intake from chronic smoking decreases cortical excitability of neurons.[71] This reduced excitability translates into inhibition of somatosensory input to the brain. Another proposed mechanism that has been shown is via chronic obstructive pulmonary disease (COPD) caused by chronic smoking. Agrawal and colleagues[72] have shown that 16.7% of COPD patients have a subclinical form of sensory peripheral neuropathy seen on electromyography studies; among these patients, it was found that those with peripheral neuropathy had a higher cigarette consumption than those patients with COPD without neuropathy. This subclinical neuropathy seems to be at risk of becoming unmasked after undergoing a PNB. COPD is a chronic state of hypoxemia, which damages peripheral nerve function in up to two-thirds of patients on electrodiagnostic studies.[73]

Preoperative neural compromise

Preoperative neural compromise can have many different causes: compressive, metabolic, toxic, ischemic, or demyelination. They may manifest as clinical or subclinical neuropathic symptoms, but regardless of whether the patient is aware of it or not, they can serve as the first insult in a phenomenon known as "double crush syndrome." It is well established that 2 low-grade insults to a nerve, whether it is in the same location or different, can be more damaging to the nerve than a single insult.[74,75]

Ischemic causes include smoking/COPD, which was previously discussed, but also encompass diabetes, vasculitis, peripheral vascular disease, and even hypertension. These comorbidities create a state of chronic ischemia, which makes nerve fibers more susceptible to any additional insult, such as a PNB.[76,77] Reported incidences of PNI following PNB in patients with diabetic neuropathy (0.4%) are higher than estimates for the general population.[78] Toxic causes would include alcohol and chemotherapy.[79] Patients with multiple sclerosis would also be at risk because of the demyelinating nature of the disease.[80,81] Compressive causes, such as cubital tunnel syndrome and carpal tunnel syndrome, are also risk factors. Regarding these chronic entrapment syndromes, it has been proposed that the PNB may simply be unmasking underlying neuropathy, which was already there before the block. There have been studies that show preexisting, asymptomatic compressive neuropathy in the contralateral elbows of patients who developed cubital tunnel syndrome after surgery.[82]

Other Factors
Surgical factors: positioning, traction, and tourniquets

Although neurologic complications from intraoperative surgical positioning and traction are not specifically related to the block procedure, it is something to keep in mind, as they can cause neurologic complications independently or exacerbate nerve injury from the block. After regional anesthesia, patients lose protective muscle tone, putting nerves at risk of compression and/or unrestricted traction during the surgery.[82,83] Low-grade stretch of peripheral nerves causes disruption of intraneural blood vessels, resulting in patchy nerve ischemia, putting these nerves at greater risk of postoperative neuropathic symptoms.[84] Padding bony prominences where superficial nerves course is also important in preventing postoperative nerve complications.[85]

The use of tourniquets has also been implicated in contributing to postoperative nerve injury.[86,87] They can cause nerve damage by compression leading to nerve ischemia. It has been well documented in the literature that a longer tourniquet time increases the chances of neurologic dysfunction.[88,89] Anderson and colleagues[19] found that patients with a higher tourniquet pressure were statistically more likely to develop neuropathic symptoms; however, the tourniquet pressure in the affected group was only 7 mm Hg greater than those without symptoms. The effectiveness of intermittent tourniquet release in preventing or mitigating neural ischemia is still debatable.[88] Using wider tourniquets, using lower cuff pressures, and limiting tourniquet time as much as possible have arisen as possible risk reduction techniques.[90]

Dexamethasone

The role of dexamethasone in conjunction with local anesthetics when performing PNBs has not been fully determined yet. An and colleagues[91] have shown that a perineural injection of dexamethasone in conjunction with bupivacaine can prolong the motor and sensory blockade in a mouse model. More interestingly, though, they also found that combining dexamethasone with bupivacaine could potentially prevent the transient neurotoxicity of bupivacaine alone. In another study, Ma and colleagues[92] showed that pretreatment of mouse neuroblastoma cells with dexamethasone before treatment with lidocaine and bupivacaine significantly diminished the bupivacaine- and lidocaine-induced cellular damage. However, a recent Cochrane review of 35 trials did not show enough evidence in the literature to determine the effectiveness of dexamethasone as an adjuvant to PNBs in lower-extremity surgery.[93] Other adjuvants, such as clonidine and midazolam, have been shown to prolong the nerve block potential of local anesthetics; however, they have not been shown to produce any kind of neuroprotective effect on nerve cells.[94]

Local Anesthetic Systemic Toxicity

LAST can be a dire consequence of unintentional intravascular injection of local anesthetic or excessive systemic absorption. In a study looking at 710,327 patients who underwent PNB, the occurrence of LAST was 1.04/1000, with only 21% of those patients experiencing a major adverse complication.[95] Although a rare occurrence, intravascular injection of high concentrations can lead to severe complications, such as hypotension, arrhythmias, cardiac arrest, grand mal seizures, and loss of consciousness.[96,97] Milder symptomatic manifestations include tinnitus, metallic taste, circumoral numbness, and agitation. The treatment is lipid emulsion administration with cardiac support. It has been shown that ultrasound guidance decreased the incidence of LAST by 65%.[77]

Infection

Infection is always a possibility with any invasive procedure when the skin barrier is broken. Given the extremely minimally invasive nature of PNBs, the risk of infection is expectedly low, especially in single-injection PNBs. In a retrospective, large-scale study looking at infections after upper- and lower-extremity ultrasound-guided single-injection PNB, Alakkad and colleagues[98] found no infections in 7476 patients. The risk of infection with an indwelling catheter after CPNB is slightly higher. The rate of catheter colonization in the literature ranges from 23% to 57%, with only 0% to 3% showing signs of local infection.[7,99–102] Coagulase-negative *Staphylococcus* is the most commonly isolated organism.[99] Some of the more severe complications reported are psoas abscesses and a single case of necrotizing fasciitis as a complication of an axillary block.[7,99,101,103] Risk factors for patients developing infected catheters have been reported as duration of catheter infusion greater than 48 hours, absence of prophylactic antibiotics, axillary or femoral catheter sites, and patients in an intensive care unit.[99]

Compartment Syndrome

PNBs have been found to be effective in pain control after acute lower-extremity fracture treatment.[11,42] There is, however, concern that a PNB may mask the earliest and most important symptom of a developing acute compartment syndrome (ACS), which is pain. Although rare, ACS can have devastating consequences if missed and is one of the most common sources of litigation against orthopedic surgeons.[104] Because of the rarity of ACS, the literature supporting or disagreeing with the use of PNBs in acute fractures and the risk of missing an ACS is limited to case reports. Of the 6 case reports available in the literature, there were only 2 cases where PNB led to a delay in diagnosis of ACS.[105] There is not enough evidence to support the use of PNBs in acute orthopedic trauma patients with long bone fractures; however, if they are used, surgeons should be vigilant and have a high suspicion for ACS.

SUMMARY

Outpatient orthopedic surgery is gradually becoming the standard across the country, as it has been found to significantly lower costs without compromising patient care.[8,106,107] Specifically in foot and ankle surgery, an outpatient total ankle replacement yields a $2500 cost savings compared with inpatient, and outpatient complex hindfoot and ankle surgery showed a 54% reduction in costs.[108,109] PNBs are largely what have made this transition possible by providing patients excellent pain control in the immediate postoperative period, allowing them to be discharged after surgery to recover in the comfort of their own home. PNBs have also been shown to decrease opioid requirements, to reduce nausea and vomiting, and to improve patient satisfaction.[3,10]

With the increasing use of PNBs, it is important to recognize that they are not without complications. The incidence of long-term nerve injury is low, generally cited as less than 1%,[19,45,48] whereas transient symptoms are higher, ranging from 0% to 41%.[17–20,48] Although rare, it is important for surgeons to discuss these potential complications with patients before surgery, as they can cause patients significant morbidity. In a retrospective review of malpractice claims related to PNBs from 2006 to 2010, Saba and colleagues[110] found that claims related to femoral blocks and popliteal blocks accounted for the second- and third-most claims, 27% and 12%, respectively. They also found that cases with the largest number of monetary settlements involved femoral and sciatic nerve blocks.

There are several ways that nerve injury can occur with PNB, including mechanical, vascular, and chemical mechanisms. There continues to be ongoing research in furthering our knowledge of how these injuries come about and ways to prevent them. Currently, ultrasound guidance seems to be the safest approach for performing PNBs and decreasing risk of LAST.[32,34] Understanding risk factors, such as preoperative neuropathy, smoking, age, and BMI, is especially important, as discussing these risk factors with patients before surgery can not only establish realistic expectations but also avoid future litigation.[111]

There is still much work to be done in ensuring that PNBs are as safe as possible for patients; however, they have been shown to be overwhelmingly successful with low overall complication rates. Future goals should include standardizing PNB procedure protocols and techniques aimed at minimizing risk of PNI, developing safe protocols for using PNBs in patients with acute lower-extremity trauma in order to avoid missing compartment syndrome, and identifying safe and effective use of adjuvants, which could improve pain control and decrease nerve damage.

CLINICS CARE POINTS

- As orthopedic surgery moves toward more and more outpatient surgery, peripheral nerve blocks are becoming standard of care in foot and ankle surgery for their effectiveness and low complication rates.

- The most common complication of peripheral nerve blocks is peripheral nerve injury, which can be caused by mechanical trauma, neurotoxic trauma, or ischemic trauma to the nerve.

- Ultrasound guidance is proven to be an effective tool for avoiding the devastating complication of local anesthetic systemic toxicity as well as increasing the success rate of nerve blocks. It has not been proven to decrease the incidence of postblock neuropathy.

- Peripheral nerve blocks should be used with caution in patients with preoperative neural compromise, as they are most at risk for developing postblock neuropathy.

- Preoperative discussion with patients should include potential complications from the nerve block.

DISCLOSURE

The authors have nothing to disclose.

REFERENCES

1. Sarrafian SK, Ibrahim IN, Breihan JH. Ankle-foot peripheral nerve block for mid and forefoot surgery. Foot Ankle 1983;4(2):86–90.
2. Pugely AJ, Martin CT, Gao Y, et al. Differences in short-term complications between spinal and general anesthesia for primary total knee arthroplasty. J Bone Joint Surg Am 2013;95(3):193–9.
3. Hadzic A, Karaca PE, Hobeika P, et al. Peripheral nerve blocks result in superior recovery profile compared with general anesthesia in outpatient knee arthroscopy. Anesth Analg 2005;100(4): 976–81.
4. Singelyn FJ, Aye F, Gouverneur JM. Continuous popliteal sciatic nerve block: an original technique to provide postoperative analgesia after foot surgery. Anesth Analg 1997;84:383–6.
5. Luiten WE, Schepers T, Luitse JS, et al. Comparison of continuous nerve block versus patient-controlled analgesia for postoperative pain and outcome after talar and calcaneal fractures. Foot Ankle Int 2014;35(11):1116–21.
6. Pakzad H, Thevendran G, Penner MJ, et al. Factors associated with longer length of hospital stay after primary elective ankle surgery for end-stage ankle arthritis. J Bone Joint Surg Am 2014; 96(1):32–9.
7. Capdevila X, Pirat P, Bringuier S, et al. Continuous peripheral nerve blocks in hospital wards after orthopedic surgery. Anesthesiology 2005;103(5): 1035–45.

8. Lovald ST, Ong KL, Malkani AL, et al. Complications, mortality, and costs for outpatient and short-stay total knee arthroplasty patients in comparison to standard-stay patients. J Arthroplasty 2014;29(3):510–5.

9. Huang A, Ryu JJ, Dervin G. Cost savings of outpatient versus standard inpatient total knee arthroplasty. Can J Surg 2017;60(1):57–62.

10. Macfarlane AJR, Prasad GA, Chan VWS, et al. Does regional anaesthesia improve outcome after total hip arthroplasty? A systematic review. Br J Anaesth 2009;103(3):335–45.

11. Elkassabany N, Cai LF, Mehta S, et al. Does regional anesthesia improve the quality of postoperative pain management and the quality of recovery in patients undergoing operative repair of tibia and ankle fractures? J Orthop Trauma 2015; 29(9):404–9.

12. Saini S, McDonald EL, Shakked R, et al. Prospective evaluation of utilization patterns and prescribing guidelines of opioid consumption following orthopedic foot and ankle surgery. Foot Ankle Int 2018;39(11):1257–65.

13. Chou LB, Wagner D, Witten DM, et al. Postoperative pain following foot and ankle surgery: a prospective study. Foot Ankle Int 2008;29(11): 1063–8.

14. Sinha A, Chan VWS. Ultrasound imaging for popliteal sciatic nerve block. Reg Anesth Pain Med 2004;29(2):130–4.

15. Brull R, McCartney CJL, Chan VWS, et al. Neurological complications after regional anesthesia: contemporary estimates of risk. Anesth Analg 2007;104(4):965–74.

16. Barrington MJ, Snyder GL. Neurologic complications of regional anesthesia. Curr Opin Anaesthesiol 2011;24(5):554–60.

17. Provenzano DA, Viscusi ER, Adams SB, et al. Safety and efficacy of the popliteal fossa nerve block when utilized for foot and ankle surgery. Foot Ankle Int 2002;23(5):394–9.

18. Borgeat A, Blumenthal S, Lambert M, et al. The feasibility and complications of the continuous popliteal nerve block: a 1001-case survey. Anesth Analg 2006;103(1):229–33.

19. Anderson JG, Bohay DR, Maskill JD, et al. Complications after popliteal block for foot and ankle surgery. Foot Ankle Int 2015;36(10):1138–43.

20. Gartke K, Portner O, Taljaard M. Neuropathic symptoms following continuous popliteal block after foot and ankle surgery. Foot Ankle Int 2012;33(4):267–74.

21. Hajek V, Dussart C, Klack F, et al. Neuropathic complications after 157 procedures of continuous popliteal nerve block for hallux valgus surgery. A retrospective study. Orthop Traumatol Surg Res 2012;98(3):327–33.

22. Emelife PI, Eng MR, Menard BL, et al. Adjunct medications for peripheral and neuraxial anesthesia. Best Pract Res Clin Anaesthesiol 2018; 32(2):83–99.

23. El-Boghdadly K, Pawa A, Chin KJ. Local anesthetic systemic toxicity: current perspectives. Local Reg Anesth 2018;11:35–44.

24. Vloka JD, Hadžić A, April E, et al. The division of the sciatic nerve in the popliteal fossa: anatomical implications for popliteal nerve blockade. Anesth Analg 2001;92(1):215–7.

25. Swenson J, Davis JJ. Anesthesia. In: Coughlin M, editor. Mann's Surgery of the Foot and Ankle. 9th edition. Chapter 5: Mosby; 2013. p. 135–51.

26. Stéfani KC, Ferreira GF, Pereira Filho MV. Postoperative analgesia using peripheral anesthetic block of the foot and ankle. Foot Ankle Int 2018; 39(2):196–200.

27. Cao X, Zhao X, Xu J, et al. Ultrasound-guided technology versus neurostimulation for sciatic nerver block: a meta-analysis. Int J Clin Exp Med 2015;8(1):273–80.

28. Abrahams MS, Aziz MF, Fu RF, et al. Ultrasound guidance compared with electrical neurostimulation for peripheral nerve block: a systematic review and meta-analysis of randomized controlled trials. Br J Anaesth 2009;102(3):408–17.

29. Munirama S, McLeod G. A systematic review and meta-analysis of ultrasound versus electrical stimulation for peripheral nerve location and blockade. Anaesthesia 2015;70(9):1084–91.

30. Gelfand HJ, Ouanes JPP, Lesley MR, et al. Analgesic efficacy of ultrasound-guided regional anesthesia: a meta-analysis. J Clin Anesth 2011;23(2):90–6.

31. Perlas A, Niazi A, McCartney C, et al. The sensitivity of motor response to nerve stimulation and paresthesia for nerve localization as evaluated by ultrasound. Reg Anesth Pain Med 2006;31(5): 445–50.

32. Sites BD, Taenzer AH, Herrick MD, et al. Incidence of local anesthetic systemic toxicity and postoperative neurologic symptoms associated with 12,668 ultrasound-guided nerve blocks: an analysis from a prospective clinical registry. Reg Anesth Pain Med 2012;37(5):478–82.

33. Barrington MJ, Watts SA, Gledhill SR, et al. Preliminary results of the Australasian Regional Anaesthesia Collaboration: a prospective audit of more than 7000 peripheral nerve and plexus blocks for neurologic and other complications. Reg Anesth Pain Med 2009;34(6):534–41.

34. Barrington MJ, Kluger R. Ultrasound guidance reduces the risk of local anesthetic systemic toxicity following peripheral nerve blockade. Reg Anesth Pain Med 2013;38(4):289–99.

35. Hadzic A, Dilberovic F, Shah S, et al. Combination of intraneural injection and high injection pressure

leads to fascicular injury and neurologic deficits in dogs. Reg Anesth Pain Med 2004;29(5):417–23.

36. Kapur E, Vuckovic I, Dilberovic F, et al. Neurologic and histologic outcome after intraneural injections of lidocaine in canine sciatic nerves. Acta Anaesthesiol Scand 2007;51(1):101–7.

37. Selander D, Brattsand R, Lundborg G, et al. Local anesthetics: importance of mode of application, concentration and adrenaline for the appearance of nerve lesions: an experimental study of axonal degeneration and barrier damage after intrafascicular injection or topical application of bupivacaine. Acta Anaesthesiol Scand 1979;23(2):127–36.

38. Rorie DK, Byer DE, Nelson DO, et al. Assessment of block of the sciatic nerve in the popliteal fossa. Anesth Analg 1980;59(5):371–6.

39. Rongstad K, Mann RA, Prieskorn D, et al. Popliteal sciatic nerve block for postoperative analgesia. Foot Ankle Int 1996;17(7):378–82.

40. Bingham AE, Fu R, Horn þJ, et al. Continuous peripheral nerve block compared with single-injection peripheral nerve block a systematic review and meta-analysis of randomized controlled trials. Reg Anesth Pain Med 2012;37(6):583–94.

41. Elliot R, Pearce CJ, Tr F, et al. Continuous infusion versus single bolus popliteal block following major ankle and hindfoot surgery: a prospective, randomized trial. Foot Ankle Int 2010;31(12):1043–7.

42. Ding DY, Manoli A III, Galos DK, et al. Continuous popliteal sciatic nerve block versus single injection nerve block for ankle fracture surgery: a prospective randomized comparative trial. J Orthop Trauma 2015;29(9):393–8.

43. Jarrell K, Mcdonald E, Shakked R, et al. Combined popliteal catheter with single-injection vs continuous-infusion saphenous nerve block for foot and ankle surgery. Foot Ankle Int 2018;39(3):332–7.

44. Auroy Y, Benhamou D, Bargues L, et al. Major complications of regional anesthesia in France: the SOS Regional Anesthesia Hotline Service. Anesthesiology 2002;97(5):1274–80.

45. Fredrickson MJ, Kilfoyle DH. Neurological complication analysis of 1000 ultrasound guided peripheral nerve blocks for elective orthopaedic surgery: a prospective study. Anaesthesia 2009;64(8):836–44.

46. Orebaugh SL, Kentor ML, Williams BA. Adverse outcomes associated with nerve stimulator-guided and ultrasound-guided peripheral nerve blocks by supervised trainees: update of a single-site database. Reg Anesth Pain Med 2012;37(6):577–82.

47. Orebaugh SL, Williams BA, Vallejo M, et al. Adverse outcomes associated with stimulator-based peripheral nerve blocks with versus without ultrasound visualization. Reg Anesth Pain Med 2009;34(3):251–5.

48. Kahn RL, Ellis SJ, Cheng J, et al. The incidence of complications is low following foot and ankle surgery for which peripheral nerve blocks are used for postoperative pain management. HSS J 2018;14:134–42.

49. Hogan QH. Pathophysiology of peripheral nerve injury during regional anesthesia. Reg Anesth Pain Med 2008;33(5):435–41.

50. Steinfeldt T, Poeschl S, Nimphius W, et al. Forced needle advancement during needle-nerve contact in a porcine model: histological outcome. Anesth Analg 2011;113(2):417–20.

51. Kerns J. The microstructure of peripheral nerves. Tech Reg Anesth Pain Manag 2008;12:127–33.

52. Selander D. Peripheral nerve injury caused by injection needles. Reg Anesth Pain Med 1993;71:323–5.

53. Selander D, Dhunér K-G, Lundborg G. Peripheral nerve injury due to injection needles used for regional anesthesia: an experimental study of the acute effects of needle point trauma. Acta Anaesthesiol Scand 1977;21(3):182–8.

54. Selander DE. Labat Lecture 2006. Regional anesthesia: aspects, thoughts, and some honest ethics; about needle bevels and nerve lesions, and back pain after spinal anesthesia. Reg Anesth Pain Med 2007;32(4):341–50.

55. Kaufman MR, Elkwood AI, Rose MI, et al. Surgical treatment of permanent diaphragm paralysis after interscalene nerve block for shoulder surgery. Anesthesiology 2013;119(2):484–7.

56. Pintaric TS, Cvetko E, Strbenc M, et al. Intraneural and perineural inflammatory changes in piglets after injection of ultrasound gel, endotoxin, 0.9% NaCl, or needle insertion without injection. Anesth Analg 2014;118(4):869–73.

57. Sturrock JE, Nunn JF. Cytotoxic effects of procaine, lignocaine and bupivacaine. Br J Anaesth 1979;51(4):273–81.

58. Gentili F, Hudson AR, Hunter D, et al. Nerve injection injury with local anesthetic agents: a light and electron microscopic, fluorescent microscopic, and horseradish peroxidase study. Neurosurgery 1980;6(3):263–72.

59. Farber SJ, Saheb-Al-Zamani M, Zieske L, et al. Peripheral nerve injury after local anesthetic injection. Anesth Analg 2013;117(3):731–9.

60. Johnson ME, Saenz JA, DaSilva AD, et al. Effect of local anesthetic on neuronal cytoplasmic calcium and plasma membrane lysis (necrosis) in a cell culture model. Anesthesiology 2002;97(6):1466–76.

61. Kitagawa N, Oda M, Totoki T. Possible mechanism of irreversible nerve injury caused by local anesthetics: detergent properties of local anesthetics and membrane disruption. Anesthesiology 2004;100(4):962–7.

62. Butterworth J, Strichartz G. Molecular mechanisms of local anesthesia: a review. Anesthesiology 1990;72(4):711–34.

63. Yang S, Abrahams MS, Hurn PD, et al. Local anesthetic Schwann cell toxicity is time and concentration dependent. Reg Anesth Pain Med 2011;36(5): 444–51.

64. Perez-Castro R, Patel S, Garavito-Aguilar ZV, et al. Cytotoxicity of local anesthetics in human neuronal cells. Anesth Analg 2009;108(3):997–1007.

65. Kalichman M. Physiologic mechanisms by which local anesthetics may cause injury to nerve and spinal cord. Reg Anesth 1993;18:448–52.

66. Myers R, Heckman H. Effects of local anesthesia on nerve blood flow: studies using lidocaine with and without epinephrine. Anesthesiology 1989; 71:757–62.

67. Ben-David B, Stahl S. Axillary block complicated by hematoma and radial nerve injury. Reg Anesth Pain Med 1999;24(1):264–6.

68. Rodríguez J, Taboada M, García F, et al. Intraneural hematoma after nerve stimulation-guided femoral block in a patient with factor XI deficiency: case report. J Clin Anesth 2011;23(3):234–7.

69. Lauf JA, Huggins P, Long J, et al. Regional nerve block complication analysis following peripheral nerve block during foot and ankle surgical procedures. Cureus 2020;12(7):1–15.

70. Nielsen KC, Guller U, Steele SM, et al. Influence of obesity on surgical regional anesthesia in the ambulatory setting: an analysis of 9,038 blocks. Anesthesiology 2005;102(1):181–7.

71. Lang N, Hasan A, Sueske E, et al. Cortical hypoexcitability in chronic smokers? A transcranial magnetic stimulation study. Neuropsychopharmacology 2008;33(10):2517–23.

72. Agrawal D, Vohra R, Gupta PP, et al. Subclinical peripheral neuropathy in stable middle-aged patients with chronic obstructive pulmonary disease. Singapore Med J 2007;48(10):887–94.

73. Gupta PP, Agarwal D. Chronic obstructive pulmonary disease and peripheral neuropathy. Lung India 2006;23:25–33.

74. Osterman A. The double crush syndrome. Orthop Clin North Am 1988;19:147–55.

75. Upton ARM, Mccomas AJ. The double crush in nerve entrapment syndromes. Lancet 1973; 302(7825):359–62.

76. Welch M, Brummett C, Welch T, et al. Perioperative peripheral nerve injuries: a retrospective study of 380,680 cases during a 10-year period at a single institution. Anesthesiology 2009;111:490–7.

77. Neal JM, Woodward CM, Harrison TK. The American Society of Regional Anesthesia and Pain Medicine checklist for managing local anesthetic systemic toxicity: 2017 version. Reg Anesth Pain Med 2018;43(2):150–3.

78. Hebl JR, Kopp SL, Schroeder DR, et al. Neurologic complications after neuraxial anesthesia or analgesia in patients with preexisting peripheral sensorimotor neuropathy or diabetic polyneuropathy. Anesth Analg 2006;103(5):1294–9.

79. Mellion M, Gilchrist JM, De La Monte S. Alcohol-related peripheral neuropathy: nutritional, toxic, or both? Muscle Nerve 2011;43(3):309–16.

80. Koff MD, Cohen JA, McIntyre JJ, et al. Severe brachial plexopathy after an ultrasound-guided single-injection nerve block for total shoulder arthroplasty in a patient with multiple sclerosis. Anesthesiology 2008;108:325–8.

81. Hebl J. Ultrasound-guided regional anesthesia and the prevention of neurologic injury: fact or fiction? Anesthesiology 2008;108(2):186–8.

82. Warner MA, Warner ME, Martin JT. Ulnar neuropathy: incidence, outcome, and risk factors in sedated or anesthetized patients. Anesthesiology 1994;81:1332–40.

83. Winfree CJ, Kline DG. Intraoperative positioning nerve injuries. Surg Neurol 2005;63(1):5–18.

84. Denny-Brown D, Doherty M. Effects of transient stretching of peripheral nerve. Arch Neurol Psych 1945;54:116–29.

85. Levy BJ, Tauberg BM, Holtzman AJ, et al. Reducing lateral femoral cutaneous nerve palsy in obese patients in the beach chair position: effect of a standardized positioning and padding protocol. J Am Acad Orthop Surg 2019;27(12):437–43.

86. Jankowski C, Keegan M, Bolton C, et al. Neuropathy following axillary brachial plexus block: is it the tourniquet? Anesthesiology 2003;99:1230–2.

87. Kornbluth ID, Freedman MK, Sher L, et al. Femoral, saphenous nerve palsy after tourniquet use: a case report. Arch Phys Med Rehabil 2003; 84(6):909–11.

88. Horlocker TT, Hebl JR, Gali B, et al. Anesthetic, patient, and surgical risk factors for neurologic complications after prolonged total tourniquet time during total knee arthroplasty. Anesth Analg 2006;102(3):950–5.

89. Jacob AK, Mantilla CB, Sviggum HP, et al. Perioperative nerve injury after total hip arthroplasty. Surv Anesthesiol 2013;57(2):94.

90. Barner KC, Landau ME, Campbell WW. A review of perioperative nerve injury to the upper extremities. J Clin Neuromuscul Dis 2003;4(3):117–23.

91. An K, Elkassabany NM, Liu J. Dexamethasone as adjuvant to bupivacaine prolongs the duration of thermal antinociception and prevents bupivacaine-induced rebound hyperalgesia via regional mechanism in a mouse sciatic nerve block model. PLoS One 2015;10(4):1–13.

92. Ma R, Wang X, Lu C, et al. Dexamethasone attenuated bupivacaine-induced neuron injury in vitro through a threonine-serine protein kinase B-

dependent mechanism. Neuroscience 2010; 167(2):329–42.

93. Pehora C, Pearson AME, Kaushal A, et al. Dexamethasone as an adjuvant to peripheral nerve block. Cochrane Database Syst Rev 2017;2017(11). https://doi.org/10.1002/14651858.CD011770.pub2.

94. Williams BA, Hough KA, Tsui BYK, et al. Neurotoxicity of adjuvants used in perineural anesthesia and analgesia in comparison with ropivacaine. Reg Anesth Pain Med 2011;36(3):225–30.

95. Rubin DS, Matsumoto MM, Weinberg G, et al. Local anesthetic systemic toxicity in total joint arthroplasty: incidence and risk factors in the United States from the national inpatient sample 1998-2013. Reg Anesth Pain Med 2018;43(2):131–7.

96. Jeng CL, Torrillo TM, Rosenblatt MA. Complications of peripheral nerve blocks. Br J Anaesth 2010;105(Suppl):i97–107.

97. Picard J, Meek T. Complications of regional anaesthesia. Anaesthesia 2010;65(Suppl 1):105–15.

98. Alakkad H, Naeeni A, Chan VWS, et al. Infection related to ultrasound-guided single-injection peripheral nerve blockade: a decade of experience at Toronto Western Hospital. Reg Anesth Pain Med 2015;40(1):82–4.

99. Capdevila X, Bringuier S, Borgeat A. Infectious risk of continuous peripheral nerve blocks. Anesthesiology 2009;110(1):182–8.

100. Cuvillon P, Ripart J, Lalourcey L, et al. The continuous femoral nerve block catheter for postoperative analgesia: bacterial colonization, infectious rate and adverse effects. Anesth Analg 2001;93(4):1045–9.

101. Neuburger M, Büttner J, Blumenthal S, et al. Inflammation and infection complications of 2285 perineural catheters: a prospective study. Acta Anaesthesiol Scand 2007;51(1):108–14.

102. Swenson JD, Bay N, Loose E, et al. Outpatient management of continuous peripheral nerve catheters

placed using ultrasound guidance: an experience in 620 patients. Anesth Analg 2006;103(6):1436–43.

103. Nseir S, Pronnier P, Soubrier S, et al. Fatal streptococcal necrotizing fasciitis as a complication of axillary brachial plexus block. Br J Anaesth 2004; 92(3):427–9.

104. Bhattacharyya T, Vrahas MS. The medical-legal aspects of compartment syndrome. J Bone Joint Surg Am 2004;86(4):864–8.

105. Tran AA, Lee D, Fassihi SC, et al. A systematic review of the effect of regional anesthesia on diagnosis and management of acute compartment syndrome in long bone fractures. Eur J Trauma Emerg Surg 2020;46(6):1281–90.

106. Lovald S, Ong K, Lau E, et al. Patient selection in outpatient and short-stay total knee arthroplasty. J Surg Orthop Adv 2014;23(1):2–8.

107. Leroux TS, Basques BA, Frank RM, et al. Outpatient total shoulder arthroplasty: a population-based study comparing adverse event and readmission rates to inpatient total shoulder arthroplasty. J Shoulder Elbow Surg 2016;25(11):1780–6.

108. Gonzalez T, Fisk E, Chiodo C, et al. Economic analysis and patient satisfaction associated with outpatient total ankle arthroplasty. Foot Ankle Int 2017;38(5):507–13.

109. Oh J, Perlas A, Lau J, et al. Functional outcome and cost-effectiveness of outpatient vs inpatient care for complex hind-foot and ankle surgery. A retrospective cohort study. J Clin Anesth 2016; 35:20–5.

110. Saba R, Brovman EY, Kang D, et al. A contemporary medicolegal analysis of injury related to peripheral nerve blocks. Pain Physician 2019;22(4):389–400.

111. Bartlett EE. Physician stress management: a new approach to reducing medical errors and liability risk. J Healthc Risk Manag 2002;22(2):3–7.

Complications Associated with the Surgical Management of Hallux Rigidus

Matthew Lunati, MD, Karim Mahmoud, MD,
Rishin Kadakia, MD, Michelle Coleman, MD/PhD,
Jason Bariteau, MD*

KEYWORDS

• Hallux rigidus • Complications • Arthrodesis • Cheilectomy • Review

---

KEY POINTS

• Surgical options can be divided between joint-sparing procedures (cheilectomy and Moberg osteotomy) and joint-sacrificing procedures (synthetic cartilage implant, interpositional arthroplasty, and arthrodesis).
• Complications associated with open cheilectomy varies greatly between 0% and 10%, with revision surgery reported at 8.8%.
• The early literature supports the use of synthetic cartilage implants with low rates of complications (<10%); however, later studies revealed less successful results with higher rates of revision and postoperative pain.
• Arthrodesis complications include malunion (6%), nonunion (0%–20%), hardware irritation, progression of arthritis involving the interphalangeal joint, and transfer metatarsalgia.

INTRODUCTION

Hallux rigidus is defined as the degenerative osteoarthritic process involving the first metatarsophalangeal (MTP) joint and is the most common arthritic pathology of the foot.[1] Like most arthritic processes, it is more prevalent in older cohorts with symptoms starting at a mean age of 51 years.[2] In the patient population greater than 50 years old, hallux rigidus has been reported to have an incidence of 2.5%.[2]

Symptoms of hallux rigidus were first described by Davies-Colley in 1887; however, there are still conflicting thoughts about the etiology of hallux rigidus.[3] Observationally, there are reported associations with metatarsus adductus, hallux valgus, and the shape of the metatarsal articular surface.[3] Patients with hallux rigidus also have a family history of this condition.[3] Hallux rigidus is a common clinical entity and treatment options depend on the severity of the disease and the functional impairments of the patient.

PATHOPHYSIOLOGY

The degenerative process associated with osteoarthritis of the knee is similar to that seen in hallux rigidus. Through the general wear and tear associated with aging, the first MTP joint becomes arthritic. There is a loss of cartilage, joint space narrowing, and osteophyte formation. Risk factors for the accelerated degeneration of this joint have been evaluated in prior literature, but no consensus exists. Coughlin and Shurnas[3] found a positive family history in two-thirds of their cohort of 110 patients with 95% of patients having bilateral disease. In this same cohort, hallux rigidus had no association with trauma, shoe wear, metatarsus primus

---

Department of Orthopaedic Surgery, Emory University School of Medicine, 59 Executive Park South, Suite 2000, Atlanta, GA 30329, USA
* Corresponding author.
E-mail address: jason.bariteau@emory.edu

Orthop Clin N Am 52 (2021) 291–296
https://doi.org/10.1016/j.ocl.2021.03.003

elevates, or Achilles tendon contracture.[3] However, hallux rigidus can also be post traumatic or associated with inflammatory arthropathies such as rheumatoid arthritis or gout.

CLINICAL PRESENTATION

Clinically, hallux rigidus presents with and insidious onset of pain located at the first MTP joint. This pain is heightened during the toe off phase of gait and typically exacerbated by shoes with heels. In the early stages of the disease, patients complain primarily of pain associated with activities requiring maximal great toe dorsiflexion, such as standing on their toes. Over time, prominent osteophytes can develop on the dorsal aspect of the metatarsal head, which can lead to irritation with shoe wear and ambulation. These dorsal osteophytes can also create pressure against the dorsomedial cutaneous nerve, causing numbness along the medial aspect of great toe.[4] As the disease progresses, gait patterns tend to be altered to off load the first MTP joint. This pattern can lead to patients complaining of lateral foot pain as they overload the lateral aspect of the foot in compensation.

On physical examination, palpable osteophytes may be tender with callous development from shoe wear. Pain tends to be elicited by passive range of motion with dorsiflexion and plantarflexion. The normal range of motion of the first MTP joint—75° of dorsiflexion and 35° of plantarflexion—is typically limited by pain.[5] The spectrum of hallux rigidus can range from pain only at the extremes of motion to pain during midrange of motion.

CLASSIFICATION SYSTEMS

There are more than 10 classification that describe the progression of hallux rigidus.[6] Outcomes are difficult to assess owing to the large number of staging systems for hallux rigidus, inconsistent use, and lack of validation between studies.[7] Most systems are organized into 3 or 4 stages and determined by a combination of radiographic parameters, clinical criteria, patient symptoms, and intraoperative findings. Three of the most used and validated systems are described in this article, namely, those described by Hatrup and Johnson, Roukis, and Coughlin and Shurnas.[7-9]

Hartrup and Johnson formulated one of the earlier classification systems in 1988, which was composed of 3 stages relevant to radiographic changes of the first MTP joint. The stages progress from 1 to 3 with increasing osteophyte development and joint space narrowing.[10] This classification system is based strictly on radiographic criteria. A criticism of this system is the lack of physical examination findings or functional deficits incorporated into the staging of hallux rigidus.[7] Radiographs alone are not enough to determine treatment options, which is a major deficiency of this grading system.

Roukis and colleagues in 2002 published the first grading system that was used in a prospective manner in a cohort consisting of 47 patients representing 50 feet.[7,9] This classification is based on a 100-point scale with allocation of 40 points for pain, 40 points for function, and 20 points for alignment and cosmesis. Criticisms of this system include use of the term exostosis to describe osteophytes and the use of metatarsus primus elevatus as a defining aspect between the grades of the classification system.[8]

One of the most used staging systems was proposed by Coughlin and colleagues in 2003. This classification consists of 5 grades (0–4),[8] which are determined by stiffness, radiographic findings of osteoarthritis, and pain with range of motion. Stage 0 is full painless range of motion with dorsiflexion to 40 to 60° and/or 10% to 20% loss of motion compared with the contralateral side, normal radiographs, and no pain, only a loss of motion and stiffness. The system progresses with grade 4 defined as less than 10° of motion and/or 75% to 100% of loss of dorsiflexion, periarticular cysts, more than one-fourth of the dorsal joint compromised, and pain at midrange of motion.[8] The distinguishing factor between grade 3 and grade 4 in this system is a clinical examination consistent with pain at the midrange of motion for grade 4 and pain only at extremes of motion for the less severe grade 3. Coughlin and colleagues' classification system was one of the first to negate metatarsus primus elevates, which has been further shown to be irrelevant to staging and outcomes of hallux rigidus.[7]

NONOPERATIVE MANAGEMENT

The initial management consists of nonoperative modalities to improve function and pain by relieving pressure at the MTP joint and dorsal osteophytes. These modalities include rocker-bottom shoe wear to limit MTP dorsiflexion, shoe wear modification to relieve dorsal pressure at the MTP joint, and activity modification.[1,11] Toe inserts are used as well to help to improve the alignment. Morton's extension orthotics can be used to help decrease pain because these orthotics offload and limit motion at the first MTP joint. When patients continue to have pain and limited function through conservative management, surgical intervention is warranted.

SURGICAL MANAGEMENT

Surgical options can be divided between joint-sparing and joint-sacrificing procedures. Joint-sparing procedures consist of cheilectomy and Moberg osteotomy. Cheilectomy and Moberg osteotomy are appropriate for patients with little radiographic evidence of first MTP joint space narrowing and subchondral sclerosis and minimal pain with range of motion.[3,9,12,13] Joint-sacrificing procedures include a synthetic cartilage implant (SCI), interpositional arthroplasty (IA), and arthrodesis. These more aggressive joint-sacrificing procedures are performed in patients with radiographic evidence of end-stage arthritis and physical examination findings of pain throughout the range of motion.[1,8,12,14–17]

Cheilectomy consists of excision and debridement of the dorsal osteophytes located on the metatarsal head along with the proximal phalanx. Intraoperatively, the dorsal third of the metatarsal head is typically sclerotic with a loss of cartilage. This dorsal aspect of the metatarsal head is removed in the cheilectomy procedure to improve the range of motion and dorsiflexion of the first MTP joint. Special attention must be taken to preserve of the collateral ligaments to prevent angular deformity.[13] Furthermore, appropriate dorsal resection is paramount, because overaggressive resection can lead to subluxation of the MTP joint.[13] Cheilectomy has been shown to have favorable outcomes with the literature revealing 75% of patients being satisfied to very satisfied with the procedure.[18]

Moberg osteotomy, or a dorsal closing wedge osteotomy of the proximal phalanx, is used to improve dorsiflexion of the first MTP joint and phalanx. The procedure consists of a closing wedge osteotomy located on the proximal aspect of the proximal phalanx of the great toe. This procedure is believed to decompress the joint and improve range of motion.[19] The improved arc of motion has been shown to translate joint contact pressure toward the plantar aspect of the first MTP joint and offload the commonly arthritic dorsal aspect of the metatarsal head.[20] The Moberg osteotomy is a reliable procedure and has demonstrated an 85% satisfaction rate.[21] The Moberg osteotomy can be performed in conjunction with a cheilectomy to further improve the range of motion with regard to dorsiflexion.

A SCI, Cartiva, was approved by the US Food and Drug Administration for the treatment of hallux rigidus and quickly gain popularity between orthopedic surgeons. The Cartiva is a molded cylinder composed of polyvinyl alcohol and saline (Wright Medical Group, Memphis, TN). It is placed into the first metatarsal head via a press–fit implantation with the help of special instrumentation with biomechanical properties similar to human hyaline cartilage. Technique includes removal of dorsal osteophytes and synovitis followed by implantation of the Cartiva, which acts as a partial spacer in the MTP joint. Pain is improved by decreased contact between arthritic joint surfaces while also preserving joint motion. Initially, outcomes revealed a neutral patient satisfaction, mild pain, and physical dysfunction,[22] but more recent studies have had conflicting evidence on implant survival and outcomes.[22–24]

IA is similar to synthetic cartilage implantation because it preserves joint mobility and function. IA combines a limited Keller resection with a biologic spacer placement made of synthetic biologic material, allograft, or autograft. Options for soft tissue interposition include tendons of the extensor digitorum, extensor hallucis brevis, gracilis, or fascia lotta, or dorsal capsule in isolation. In patients that prefer to maintain joint motion, IA has been shown to have improved patient outcomes postoperatively.[25]

Arthrodesis is the gold standard for the treatment for end-stage arthritis of the first MTP joint. Many techniques have been described to achieve appropriate fusion consisting of plates, screws, wires, and staples. The most commonly used fusion technique is a combination of a dorsal plate with a lag screw, which has been shown to be the most stable construct.[26] The optimum position for fusion of the first MTP joint is in 5° to 15° of valgus and 10° to 20° of dorsiflexion with neutral rotation.[19] Outcomes after arthrodesis include reliable relief of pain while only minimally decreasing range of motion in joint with baseline stiffness.[8,9,12,15,27–29] Despite the loss of motion at the first MTP joint, patients continue to be very active, with limited functional loss. Studies examining the outcomes after first MTP joint arthrodesis have demonstrated that even young patients can get back to being active and playing sports with limited functional consequences.[30]

COMPLICATIONS OF HALLUX RIGIDUS SURGERY
Cheilectomy
Cheilectomy is a relatively safe procedure with a low risk profile. Sidon and colleagues[18] reported

on the long-term outcomes after dorsal cheilectomy in 165 patients with a mean follow-up of 6.6 years, which showed 5% underwent subsequent surgery. Most complications can be attributed to technical errors in the osteotomy, either removing too much bone to cause subluxation, not removing enough (which leads to continued pain), or destabilizing the joint during dissection.[31] The complication rates are much higher with newer, more minimally invasive techniques for performing cheilectomy.[32]

Complications associated with open cheilectomy vary greatly between 0% and 8% in a systematic review looking at the need for revision surgery after isolated cheilectomy.[33] Injury to the dorsal medial cutaneous nerve has been shown to occur at a rate of 8.9% and delayed wound healing at 6.5%.[33] Dorsal exostosis recurrence after cheilectomy has been shown to be as high as 30% in long-term follow-up.[34] Revision surgery was reported at 8.8% by a systematic review done by Roukis and colleagues[33] with revision arthrodesis as the most common revision surgery performed. Rarely, avascular necrosis of the metatarsal head occurs after cheilectomy. This outcome may be associated with an overly aggressive release of collateral and plantar structures to gain motion; therefore, attention must be given to preserve the plantar lateral blood supply of the metatarsal head during the procedure. Overall, cheilectomy has been shown to have successful outcomes with low rates of complications.

MOBERG OSTEOTOMY

Moberg osteotomy is often performed in conjunction with either cheilectomy or Cartiva. A paucity of literature exists on the rates of complications associated with Moberg osteotomy because it is a procedure rarely done in isolation. However, complications include nonunion, varus or valgus malunion, symptomatic hardware, and intraarticular extension of the osteotomy.[35] The most common revision surgery for Moberg osteotomy is arthrodesis for continuous pain, at 5%.[21]

SYNTHETIC CARTILAGE IMPLANTS

SCIs, like Cartiva, have had a controversial role in the treatment of hallux rigidus. Initially, Baumhauer and colleagues,[36] in 2016, organized a multicenter prospective, randomized noninferiority study evaluating outcome measures after SCI versus first MTP arthrodesis. This study included 152 patients with SCI and 50 arthrodesis and used a visual analogue scale pain score and the Foot and Ankle Ability Measure sport scale to highlight equivalent pain relief and function outcomes between the 2 procedures. At 2 years, the SCI cohort was found to have a 9% revision to arthrodesis rate. This cohort was evaluated again at 5 years, and more than 90% of the patients with SCI were found to have further improvements in pain and function.[37] Furthermore, they found 7.6% of patients underwent conversion to arthrodesis from years 2 to 5.

Despite the early literature in support of the use of SCI, later studies revealed less successful results with higher rates of revision and postoperative pain. Cassinelli and associates[22] evaluated the early outcomes and complications of SCIs in 64 feet and 60 patients. They found a 20% reoperation rate, most commonly conversion to arthrodesis owing to continued postoperative pain. The main reason for persistent pain after Cartiva implantation includes pain related to subsidence, breakage of the implant, or the development of a foreign body reaction.[38] More recently, Chrea and colleagues[23] compared clinical outcomes of 166 patients undergoing cheilectomy and Moberg osteotomy with insertion of an SCI (72 patients) and those without an SCI (94 patients). Within the SCI cohort, they found most common complications to be revision (5%), persistent pain (11.7%), and infection (5%).[23] Although evidence exists in support of the use of SCI, there are conflicting rates of complications and rates of revision surgery owing to continued postoperative pain.

INTERPOSITION ARTHROPLASTY

Retrospective reviews evaluating IA report complications of metatarsalgia, weakness of hallux, diminished push off, and loss of ground contact of great toe.[25,39,40] Lau and colleagues[39] performed a retrospective review of 19 patients, including 24 feet, and found high complication rate within the IA cohort.[39] Hallux weakness was seen in 72.7% of these patients. They also found greater weight transfer to lesser metatarsal heads through pedobarographic analysis with IA.[39]

ARTHRODESIS

Complications associated with MTP fusion are most frequently associated with technical factors by the surgeon: nonunion and malunion.[1,19] Other complications include hardware irritation, progression of arthritis involving the interphalangeal joint, and transfer metatarsalgia.[27] Correct positioning of the hallux for fusion in both the coronal and sagittal plane is paramount. Overall incidence of malunion has been shown to be as high as 6.1%, with dorsiflexion malunion accounting for 87.1%.[41] An overly dorsiflexed fused great toe can lead to abutment of the toe into shoe wear, leading to subungual hematoma. Also, excessive dorsiflexion can result in overload of the first metatarsal and sesamoids causing pain. Coronally, fusion in excessive abduction can lead to friction and skin breakdown between the first and second toes. Adduction leads to varus and difficulty with shoe wear. Nonunion rates after a first MTP arthrodesis varies in literature between 0% and 20%.[41] Critical factors for union include appropriate joint preparation and adequate fixation. Despite the loss of range of motion associated with arthrodesis, complication rates are low with appropriate joint preparation and outcomes are favorable.

SUMMARY

Multiple surgical techniques have been developed for the treatment of hallux rigidus. The literature reveals good outcomes following cheilectomy with or without Moberg osteotomy and arthrodesis with low complication rates. Conflicting evidence exists for SCIs and IA for both outcomes and complications associated with these 2 procedures. Common complications associated with all surgical interventions are wound complications and technical error. Despite these complications, appropriate surgical interventions for grades of hallux rigidus have high levels of patient satisfaction.

CLINICS CARE POINTS

- Joint sparing and joint sacrificing procedures have successful outcomes
- Cheilectomy has been shown to have 75% satisfaction rate
- Arthrodesis has been shown to have no decrease in function post operatively
- Common complications include wound breakdown and technical error
- Complications following cheilectomy are most related to technical errors including removal of too much bone resulting in subluxation, or destabilizing the joint during dissection
- Nonunion after arthrodesis can be improved with adequate joint preparation

---

DISCLAIMERS

No author, their immediate family, or any research foundation with which they are affiliated received any financial payments or other benefits from any commercial entity related to the subject of this article.

REFERENCES

1. Deland JT, Williams BR. Surgical management of hallux rigidus. J Am Acad Orthop Surg 2012;20: 347–58.
2. Gould N, Schneider W, Ashikaga T. Epidemiological survey of foot problems in the continental United States: 1978-1979. Foot Ankle 1980;1:8–10.
3. Coughlin MJ, Shurnas PS. Hallux rigidus: demographics, etiology, and radiographic assessment. Foot Ankle Int 2003;24:731–43.
4. Keiserman LS, Sammarco VJ, Sammarco GJ. Surgical treatment of the hallux rigidus. Foot Ankle Clin 2005;10:75–96.
5. Shereff MJ, Bejjani FJ, Kummer FJ. Kinematics of the first metatarsophalangeal joint. J Bone Joint Surg Am 1986;68:392–8.
6. Dillard S, Schilero C, Chiang S, et al. Intra- and interobserver reliability of three classification systems for hallux rigidus. J Am Podiatr Med Assoc 2018. https://doi.org/10.7547/16-126.
7. Beeson P, Phillips C, Corr S, et al. Classification systems for hallux rigidus: a review of the literature. Foot Ankle Int 2008;29:407–14.
8. Coughlin MJ, Shurnas PS. Hallux rigidus. Grading and long-term results of operative treatment. J Bone Joint Surg Am 2003;85:2072–88.
9. Roukis TS, Jacobs PM, Dawson DM, et al. A prospective comparison of clinical, radiographic, and intraoperative features of hallux rigidus. J foot Ankle Surg 2002;41:76–95.
10. Hattrup SJ, Johnson KA. Subjective results of hallux rigidus following treatment with cheilectomy. Clin Orthop Relat Res 1988;(226):182–91.
11. Kunnasegaran R, Thevendran G. Hallux rigidus: nonoperative treatment and orthotics. Foot Ankle Clin 2015;20:401–12.
12. Anderson MR, Ho BS, Baumhauer JF. Current concepts review: hallux rigidus. Foot Ankle Orthop 2018;3. 2473011418764461.
13. Heller WA, Brage ME. The effects of cheilectomy on dorsiflexion of the first metatarsophalangeal joint. Foot Ankle Int 1997;18:803–8.
14. Chraim M, Bock P, Alrabai HM, et al. Long-term outcome of first metatarsophalangeal joint fusion in the treatment of severe hallux rigidus. Int Orthop 2016;40:2401–8.
15. Fuhrmann RA. First metatarsophalangeal arthrodesis for hallux rigidus. Foot Ankle Clin 2011;16:1–12.

16. Kumar S, Pradhan R, Rosenfeld PF. First metatarso-phalangeal arthrodesis using a dorsal plate and a compression screw. Foot Ankle Int 2010;31: 797–801.

17. Lam A, Chan JJ, Surace MF, et al. Hallux rigidus: how do I approach it? World J Orthop 2017;8: 364–71.

18. Sidon E, Rogero R, Bell T, et al. Long-term follow-up of cheilectomy for treatment of hallux rigidus. Foot Ankle Int 2019;40:1114–21.

19. Galois L, Hemmer J, Ray V, et al. Surgical options for hallux rigidus: state of the art and review of the literature. Eur J Orthop Surg Traumatol 2020; 30:57–65.

20. Kim PH, Chen X, Hillstrom H, et al. Moberg osteotomy shifts contact pressure plantarly in the first metatarsophalangeal joint in a biomechanical model. Foot Ankle Int 2016;37:96–101.

21. O'Malley MJ, Basran HS, Gu Y, et al. Treatment of advanced stages of hallux rigidus with cheilectomy and phalangeal osteotomy. J Bone Joint Surg Am 2013;95:606–10.

22. Cassinelli SJ, Chen S, Charlton TP, et al. Early outcomes and complications of synthetic cartilage implant for treatment of hallux rigidus in the United States. Foot Ankle Int 2019;40:1140–8.

23. Chrea B, Eble SK, Day J, et al. Comparison between polyvinyl alcohol implant and cheilectomy with Moberg osteotomy for hallux rigidus. Foot Ankle Int 2020;41:1031–40.

24. An TW, Cassinelli S, Charlton TP, et al. Radiographic and magnetic resonance imaging of the symptomatic synthetic cartilage implant. Foot Ankle Int 2020;41:25–30.

25. Roukis TS. Outcome following autogenous soft tissue interpositional arthroplasty for end-stage hallux rigidus: a systematic review. J foot Ankle Surg 2010; 49:475–8.

26. Politi J, John H, Njus G, et al. First metatarsal-phalangeal joint arthrodesis: a biomechanical assessment of stability. Foot Ankle Int 2003;24:332–7.

27. DeSandis B, Pino A, Levine DS, et al. Functional outcomes following first metatarsophalangeal arthrodesis. Foot Ankle Int 2016;37:715–21.

28. van Doeselaar DJ, Heesterbeek PJ, Louwerens JW, et al. Foot function after fusion of the first metatarsophalangeal joint. Foot Ankle Int 2010;31:670–5.

29. Lunati MP, Manz WJ, Maidman SD, et al. Effect of age on complication rates and outcomes following first metatarsophalangeal arthrodesis for hallux rigidus. Foot Ankle Int 2020;41:1347–54.

30. Da Cunha RJ, MacMahon A, Jones MT, et al. Return to sports and physical activities after first metatarsophalangeal joint arthrodesis in young patients. Foot Ankle Int 2019;40:745–52.

31. Coughlin MJ, Shurnas PS. Hallux rigidus: surgical techniques (cheilectomy and arthrodesis). JBJS 2004;86:119–30.

32. Stevens R, Bursnall M, Chadwick C, et al. Comparison of complication and reoperation rates for minimally invasive versus open cheilectomy of the first metatarsophalangeal joint. Foot Ankle Int 2020; 41:31–6.

33. Roukis TS. The need for surgical revision after isolated cheilectomy for hallux rigidus: a systematic review. J foot Ankle Surg 2010;49:465–70.

34. Easley ME, Davis WH, Anderson RB. Intermediate to long-term follow-up of medial-approach dorsal cheilectomy for hallux rigidus. Foot Ankle Int 1999;20:147–52.

35. Citron N, Neil M. Dorsal wedge osteotomy of the proximal phalanx for hallux rigidus. Long-term results. J Bone Joint Surg Br 1987;69:835–7.

36. Baumhauer JF, Singh D, Glazebrook M, et al. Prospective, randomized, multi-centered clinical trial assessing safety and efficacy of a synthetic cartilage implant versus first metatarsophalangeal arthrodesis in advanced hallux rigidus. Foot Ankle Int 2016;37:457–69.

37. Glazebrook M, Blundell CM, O'Dowd D, et al. Midterm outcomes of a synthetic cartilage implant for the first metatarsophalangeal joint in advanced hallux rigidus. Foot Ankle Int 2019;40:374–83.

38. Mahmoud K, Metikala S, Mehta SD, et al. The Role of Weightbearing Computed Tomography Scan in Hallux Valgus. Foot Ankle Int 2020. https://doi.org/10.1177/1071100720962398. 1071100720962398.

39. Lau JT, Daniels TR. Outcomes following cheilectomy and interpositional arthroplasty in hallux rigidus. Foot Ankle Int 2001;22:462–70.

40. Coughlin MJ, Shurnas PJ. Soft-tissue arthroplasty for hallux rigidus. Foot Ankle Int 2003;24:661–72.

41. Roukis TS. Nonunion after arthrodesis of the first metatarsal-phalangeal joint: a systematic review. J foot Ankle Surg 2011;50:710–3.

Moving?

Make sure your subscription moves with you!

To notify us of your new address, find your **Clinics Account Number** (located on your mailing label above your name), and contact customer service at:

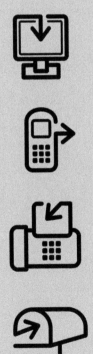

Email: journalscustomerservice-usa@elsevier.com

800-654-2452 (subscribers in the U.S. & Canada)
314-447-8871 (subscribers outside of the U.S. & Canada)

Fax number: 314-447-8029

Elsevier Health Sciences Division
Subscription Customer Service
3251 Riverport Lane
Maryland Heights, MO 63043

ELSEVIER

Printed and bound by CPI Group (UK) Ltd, Croydon, CR0 4YY

08/05/2025

01864713-0012